Cambridge Elements ≡

Elements in Ancient East Asia
edited by
Erica Fox Brindley
Pennsylvania State University
Rowan Kimon Flad
Harvard University

MEDICINE AND HEALING IN ANCIENT EAST ASIA

A View from Excavated Texts

Constance A. Cook
Lehigh University

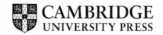

CAMBRIDGE
UNIVERSITY PRESS

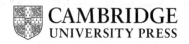

Shaftesbury Road, Cambridge CB2 8EA, United Kingdom

One Liberty Plaza, 20th Floor, New York, NY 10006, USA

477 Williamstown Road, Port Melbourne, VIC 3207, Australia

314–321, 3rd Floor, Plot 3, Splendor Forum, Jasola District Centre,
New Delhi – 110025, India

103 Penang Road, #05–06/07, Visioncrest Commercial, Singapore 238467

Cambridge University Press is part of Cambridge University Press & Assessment,
a department of the University of Cambridge.

We share the University's mission to contribute to society through the pursuit of
education, learning and research at the highest international levels of excellence.

www.cambridge.org
Information on this title: www.cambridge.org/9781108972208

DOI: 10.1017/9781108975834

When citing this work, please include a reference to the DOI 10.1017/9781108975834

First published 2023

A catalogue record for this publication is available from the British Library.

ISBN 978-1-108-97220-8 Paperback
ISSN 2632-7325 (online)
ISSN 2632-7317 (print)

Medicine and Healing in Ancient East Asia

A View from Excavated Texts

Elements in Ancient East Asia

DOI: 10.1017/9781108975834
First published online: June 2023

Constance A. Cook
Lehigh University
Author for correspondence: Constance A. Cook, cac8@lehigh.edu

Abstract: This Element first discusses the creation of transmitted medical canons that are generally dated from early imperial times through to the medieval era and then, by way of contrast, provides translations and analyses of non-transmitted texts from the pre-imperial late Shang and Zhou eras and the early imperial Qin and Han eras, as well as a brief discussion covering the period through the eleventh-century CE. The Element focuses on the evolution of concepts, categories of illness, and diagnostic and treatment methodologies evident in the newly discovered material and reveals a side of medical practice not reflected in the canons. It is both traditions of healing – the canons and the currents of local practice revealed by these texts – that influenced the development of East Asian medicine more broadly. The local practices show there was no real evolution from magical to non-magical medicine. This title is also available as Open Access on Cambridge Core.

Keywords: ancient, China, medicine, magical, cosmic

ISBNs: 9781108972208 (PB), 9781108975834 (OC)
ISSNs: 2632-7325 (online), 2632-7317 (print)

Contents

1 Introduction

This Element first discusses the creation of transmitted medical canons that are generally dated from early imperial times through to the medieval era and then, by way of contrast, provides translations and analyses of non-transmitted texts from the pre-imperial late Shang (ca. 1200 BCE–1045 BCE) and Zhou (1045 BCE–221 BCE) eras and the early imperial Qin (221 BCE–206 BCE) and Han (206 BCE–220 CE) eras, as well as a brief discussion covering the period through the eleventh century CE. The Element focuses on the evolution of concepts, categories of illness, and diagnostic and treatment methodologies evident in the newly discovered material and reveals a side of medical practice not reflected in the canons. It is both traditions of healing —the canons edited by literati and the currents of local practice revealed by these texts – that influenced the development of East Asian medicine more broadly.

The earliest texts, written on bones, originate from the Yellow River (Huang He) Valley. The next set, dated as early as the fourth century BCE and as late as the tenth century CE, and written on bamboo, silk, and eventually paper, were pre-served in anaerobic tombs in the Yangzi River Valley and Sichuan Basin and the dry desert caves and sites in Gansu. The local practices reflected in these texts make evident that there was no real evolution from magical to non-magical medicine. The rational ur-scientific approach to the body as a system of meridians and viscera powered by "natural" forces such as the variant modes of *qi* 氣 ("breath, air, life energy") – *yin* and *yang* 陰陽 (dark and light, negative and positive) and *wuxing* 五行 (the Five Agents: Wood, Water, Metal, Fire, and Earth) – that were so basic to canonical knowledge was not universally applied. Only during the early imperial age (the second century BCE through to the fifth century CE) did a vision of the inner body as a system of channels pulsating with these modes of *qi* emerge. These *mai* 脈 ("vessels") or *jingluo* 經絡 ("channel network, conduits, meridians") were also only slowly connected to a set of inner spaces called the *wuzang liufu* 五臟六腑 (the Five Storage Depots or Viscera and the Six Cavities: Heart, Lungs, Liver, Spleen, Kidneys and Gall Bladder, Stomach, Large and Small Intestines, Bladder, and *san jiao*, or "the Triple Burners") (Lo, 2018b). Yet these spaces, largely unacknowledged in the earliest layers of the non-transmitted literature, became fundamental to later canon-based medical practice. Evidence for diagnostic methodologies such as pulse-taking and treatments such as moxibustion and acupuncture, which were key to the later system, is also scarce.

2 Transmitted Medical Knowledge and the Creation of Canons

The primary medical canon for East Asian medicine is the *Inner Classic of the Yellow Emperor* (*Huangdi Neijing* 黃帝內經, hereafter *HDNJ*), which accord-ing to tradition can be traced back to a prehistorical sage, though scholars now suggest it was mostly Tang (618–907 CE) material edited by Song period literati (960–1279 CE) and may or may not preserve textual threads traceable back to the early imperial era (Keegan, 1988; Sivin, 1993; Harper, 1998). Two books exist – separately called *Suwen* 素問 (*Plain Questions*, focusing on cosmological theory) and *Lingshu* 靈樞 (*Divine Pivot*, focusing on acupuncture therapy). Two other books include one reconstructed text (*Taisu* 太素) and one lost text that is mentioned in later texts (*Mingtang* 明堂, short for *Mingtang kongxue zhenjiu zhiyao* 明堂孔穴鍼灸治要 or *Huangdi mingtang jing*). Transmitted medical literature, contingent so often on the whims of political sponsorship or teacher–student relationships, is by nature subject to the successive hands of editors and archivists.

Hints of the original diversity of archives and private libraries are appearing now in the counternarratives preserved in newly discovered texts. Dating from the second millennium BCE to the tenth century CE, fragmentary and complete manuscripts show both a long history of magical practices used for healing and the continued integration of evolved forms of these practices with the more cosmologically based medical ideologies advocated by *HDNJ* (Harper, 1998, 1999b, 2005; Strickmann, 2002; Cook, 2006, 2013b). That is, we can now read from a new perspective the medical classics that scholar-physicians had continued to edit, refine, and debate (Brown, 2015, 96; Lo, 2018, 590–591).

The classics tend to emphasize the role of natural cosmological agencies, the modes of *qi* that influenced both health and illness within the human body, and the outer layered world of geographical, social, and celestial spaces. Human emotion was an internally generated type of *qi* affecting and affected by the other modes of *qi* (Hsu, 2008–9). The movement of or change in these modes was regulated by the numerology of time: the seasons, the ritual sexagenary calendar, months, days, and hours (Lo, 2018, 590; Lo & Gu, in press). This medicine of systemic correspondence, as termed by Paul Unschuld (1985), is often distinguished by scholars from magical or demonic medicine, but in practice the two overlapped.

Famous Men and Cosmic Medicine

The first half of the Han dynasty, known as the Western Han dynasty (206 BCE–9 CE), was a time of long-lived emperors, vast territorial claims, and the consolidation of philosophical and technical knowledge. There is a tendency during this era to link the development of medical knowledge to legendary sages, such as Huangdi (the Yellow Emperor) (Lo, 2018, 577–578, 587). In fact, most ancient medical works, transmitted or not, have no definite author or obvious context of compilation, a situation the *HDNJ* shares with the *Classic of Difficult*

Issues (*Nanjing* 難經, also known as the *Huangdi bashiyi nanjing* 皇帝八十一難經), probably first compiled in the latter or Eastern Han period (206 BCE–220 CE) (Lo & Li, 2007; Unschuld, 2016b, 25–26). Non-transmitted materials rarely have titles, much less any known authorship. Most titles are assigned by modern scholars based on assumptions of textual classification.

Many canons were lost and exist only in reconstructed forms (Keegan 1988; Sivin, 1993; Unschuld, 2016a, 22–25). The *Shanghan zabing lun* 傷寒雜病論 written by Zhang Ji 張機 (142–220?; also known as Zhang Zhongjing 張仲景) had been lost but was later reconstructed by Wang Shuhe 王叔和 (210–85; also known as Wang Xi 熙) into two foundational texts: *Cold Damage Treatise* (*Shanghan lun* 傷寒論) and *Essential Prescriptions of the Golden Cabinet* (*Jingui yaolüe* 金櫃要略) (Zhang Ji, 2013, 2014). Notably, the key concepts of these early imperial texts, such as illness from external *qi* modes, known as "perverse *qi*" (*xie qi* 邪氣) in the canons, such as "wind" (*feng* 風), "heat" (*re* 熱), and "cold" (*han* 寒), only begin to appear in the non-transmitted texts – some even titled – from the Sichuan Basin, in a tomb dated to around 188 BCE in Laoguanshan 老官山 (Tianhui 天回, Chengdu, Sichuan) (not yet formally published; hereafter LGS). Even so, these elements of newer medicine were mixed with practices centuries old.

Early canons focused on treatments not evident in early non-transmitted literature, such as "acumoxa" (*zhenjiu* 鍼灸, the treatment of *qi* vessels at specific points on the body with needles or burning cones). An example, compiled out of earlier texts by Huangfu Mi 皇甫謐 (214–82), was published as the *Classic of A and B* (*Jiayi jing* 甲乙經, also known by various names such as *Huangdi jiayi jing* and *Zhenjiu jiayi jing*). The earliest version of this text is from the Ming dynasty (1368–1644). On the other hand, non-transmitted sources may attest to the influential *Vessel Classic* (*Maijing* 脈經) by Wang Shuhe, also compiled from earlier sources. These include a text self-titled the *Vessel Document* (*Maishu* 脈書) found in a 186 BCE tomb in Zhangjiashan 張家山 (ZJS) (Jiangling, Hubei) and the various vessel and cauterization texts discovered in a 168 BCE tomb at Mawangdui 馬王堆 (MWD) (Changsha, Hunan). An MWD text, which modern scholars call *Model of the Vessels* (*Maifa* 脈法), preserves parts of the earlier *Vessel Document* from ZJS (Harper, 1998, 22–24, 30–32). Notably, there is little to no evidence for acumoxa in either text.

When did the literati who compiled the canons begin to frame their healing methods as sourced from ancient sages? Non-transmitted texts reveal the device as early as the fourth century BCE, but records of lost texts in transmitted histories also reveal the trend, though with different sets of sages and a vast array of genres. The late Han historian Ban Gu 班固 (32–92 CE), incorporating work by the Han physician Li Zhuguo 李柱國, listed books in the bibliographic section ("Yiwen zhi" 藝文志) of the *Documents of Han* (*Han shu* 漢書) according to thematic categories (Hunter, 2018, 763). Huangdi, a progenitor popularized in the Han dynasty, is associated with texts in a number of categories, such as Daoist practices and ideology, *yin* and *yang*, orally transmitted stories, astronomy (and astrology), *wuxing* (the Five Agents), calendars, various types of divination, medical classics (*yi jing* 醫經), canonized recipes (*jingfang* 經方, decoctions of herbs, minerals, insects, and other substances), sexual methods (*fangzhong* 房中), and techniques for spiritual transcendence (*shenxian* 神僊). Another popular Han sage, the Divine Husbandman (Shennong 神農), associated traditionally with herbal medicine, is linked to books in the categories of agriculture, *yin* and *yang*, *wuxing*, various divination methods, recipes, and spiritual transcendence. Just as the Huangdi tradition spurred the development of later classics focusing on vessel theory and acupuncture (such as the *Jiayi jing*), the Shennong tradition inspired collections of pharmaceutical recipes and led the occult alchemist Tao Hongjing 陶宏景 (456–536) to formalize the study of *bencao* 本草 or *materia medica* (Brown, 2015, 8; Bian, 2020, 6).

The roots of Han cosmic medicine and the framing devices are found in late Zhou manuscripts, mostly dating to the fourth century BCE. As in the *HDNJ*, knowledge transmission is through a question-and-answer format, with the senior authority figure guided by sage advisors. In the recently discovered bamboo texts presently preserved by Tsinghua University, we find that instead of the *HDNJ* paradigm of Huangdi as the avatar for political authority and Qi Bo 歧伯 (among others) as the technical expert, the paradigmatic pair were the mythical founder of the Shang dynasty, Tang 湯 (also known as Chengtang 成湯), and Yi Yin 伊尹, the wise minister. Both Tang and Yi Yin appear in a number of Tsinghua texts; they are well known in received literature (Tang goes by various names, [Feng Yicheng 2019, 74–75]; and Yi Yin is a sage advisor but also a magician, a shaman, and a cook, [Allan 2015]) and may appear in paleographical texts as early as the Shang oracle bones (Li, Ai, & Lü, 2019). Neither Tang nor Yi Yin feature in Ban Gu's list. According to commentators and later scholars, sages such as Huangdi and Shennong understood the cosmos and thus legitimized the authority of the text (Bian, 2020, 32, 81).

The range of topics linked by Ban Gu to healing reveals early literati approaches to cosmic medicine. *Wuxing* is explained as the five constant forms of *qi* (五行者, 五常之形氣也), which guide everything from human affairs to the movement of the stars. "Masters of recipes listed in canons" (*jing fangzhe* 經方者) are defined as:

[Specialists who] relied on the cold and warm qualities of herbs and minerals [in concert with] the shallow and deep [pulse] measurements of illness to determine the density of herbal flavors appropriate to the *qi* reaction; [they] distinguished the five types of Bitter and six types of Pungent, providing the doses of Water and Fire [necessary] to penetrate the closed-off areas and release those knotted areas [in the bodies of the patients] in order to revert them back to normal.

本草石之寒溫, 量疾病之淺深, 假藥味之滋, 因氣感之宜, 辯五苦六辛, 致水火之齊, 以通閉解結, 反之於平.

If the recipes were inappropriate, causing too much heat or cold and resulting in "inner damage of the *jing* 精 (vital essence, spirit) and *qi*" (*jing qi neishang* 精氣內傷), then, even though the damage was not outwardly apparent, a physician (*yi* 醫) had to be consulted. The section on "those proficient in the medical canon" (*yijingzhe* 醫經者) notes that:

[They] base the categorization of the 100 illnesses on the human indicators of blood vessels, the conduit system, bones and marrow, *yin* and *yang*; [they] separate the living from the dead and with the use of the [pulse] measurement, the needling stone, decoctions, and fire (cauterization), [they] determine the appropriately balanced blend of the 100 herbs.

原人血脈經絡骨髓陰陽表裏, 以起百病之本, 死生之分, 而用度箴石湯火所施, 調百藥齊和之所宜.

Here, we see from Ban Gu's perspective three levels of diagnosis and treatment. First, "illness" or the "ailment, disorder, disease" (*bing* 病) is determined by "indicators" (*biao* 表) revealed through pulse measurements of the *yin*-and-*yang* values in the vessels of blood (*xue* 血) and of *qi*, as well as indicators in the skeletal structure. Notably, the treatment involves a stone "needle" and cauterization rather than acupuncture and moxibustion, along with herbal recipes. The MWD manuscripts dating to the second century BCE attest to an early science of pulse-reading, cauterization, and decoctions but not to needling, although lancing stones (*bian*) existed earlier and metal needles, possibly medical, were found in slightly later tombs in Guangxi and Hebei (Harper, 1998, 5, 92; Lan Riyong, 1993; Zhongguo shehui kexueyuan kaogu yanjiusuo 1980, vol. 1, fig. 78).

Several centuries after Ban Gu, Huangfu Mi summarized his understanding of the creation of Chinese medicine and treatment methods in the *Classic of A and B* (translation adapted from Brown [2015, 98]; Huang-fu Mi, 1994, xix):

As for the rise of the Way of Medicine, it has been around for a long time. In High Antiquity, the Divine Husbandman (Shennong) first understood the 100 medicines by tasting plants. Huangdi consulted with followers, Qibo, Bogao

伯高, and Shaoyu 少俞, about how to evaluate the five viscera and six cavities (*wuzang liufu*) on the inside and to synthesize the symptoms of conduits of blood and *qi* from appearances on the outside. [They] triangulated [this information] with the [cosmic indicators] of the Sky and Earth and with the basic natures of what they examined in human and other [sensate] beings, [seeing that] when the spirit [of *yang*] was exhausted, [the *qi*] pivots and changes [to *yin*], so the Way of Needling arose thereby. Their treatises were miraculous; the Thunder Lord (Leigong 雷公) received them and passed them on to talents like Yi Yin, who edited and made decoctions from *Divine Husbandman's Materia Medica* (*Shenong bencao*).

夫醫道所興, 其來久矣. 上古神農始嘗草木而知百藥. 黃帝諮訪岐伯, 伯高, 少俞之徒, 內考五臟六腑, 外綜經絡血氣色候, 參之天地, 驗之人物, 本性命, 窮神極變, 而針道生焉. 其論至妙, 雷公受業傳之於後. 伊尹以亞聖之才, 撰用 "神農本草" 以為湯液.

Interestingly, the Thunder Lord is mentioned instead of Tang in combination with Yi Yin. Rather than dialogues between sage kings and magical ministers, Huangfu categorizes the development of medical diagnostic and treatment methods by medical lineages. He lists later sage-like healers, such as the famed practitioners of pulse diagnostics and acumoxa therapy, the presumed late fifth-century BCE Bian Que 扁鵲 (Qin Yueren 秦越人) and the second-century BCE Cang Gong 倉公 (Chunyu Yi 淳于意), who are mentioned in Han sources but who left no written legacies (Brown, 2015, 41–86; Hsu, 2010, 3–4; although scholars link some of the LGS texts to Bian Que: Du Feng, 2014b). Methods linked to these healers, such as examining or palpating vessels (*zhen mai* 診脈 or *qie mai* 切), needling (*ci* 刺), cauterizing (*jiu* 灸), and decoctions (*tang* 湯), cannot be confirmed before the second century BCE (Hsu, 2010, 4, 10). Huangfu credits his predecessors, including those closer to his own time, such as Zhang Zhongjing (Zhang Ji), the author of the influential *Cold Damage Treatise*, and Hua Tuo 華佗 (d. 208 CE), a healer known for his early surgical techniques (Brown, 2015, 99, 101, 158–159). Manuscripts confirm that knowledge later consolidated by Zhong Ji and Huangfu Mi derived from numerous sources.

Early imperial manuscripts reveal a long tradition of treating the same ailments diagnosed by pulse-reading with recipes (*fang* 方). The ingredients were made into soups, pressed onto the body, ground up into warmed alcohol, or made into pills. They are often combined with magical formulas, prayers, invocations, and exorcistic choreographies. The blurring of *materia medica* with magic is reflected in the early pharmaceutical canon by the Daoist master Ge Hong 葛洪 (281–341), the author of the eponymous *Master Who Embraces Simplicity* (*Baopuzi* 抱朴子). Such chapters as "Transcendent Medicines"

("Xianyao" 仙藥) reflect the blending of "nurturing life" (*yangsheng* 養生) practices for achieving a long life with local healing practices (see the diagram showing the relationship of healing the sick and attaining transcendence through the modulated use of toxic drugs in Liu, 2021, 5). Medical canons attributed to Ge Hong include the *Recipes from Behind the Elbow (in the Sleeve) to Rescue the Dying* (*Zhouhou qiuzu fang* 肘後求卒方), which survives only in a version edited by the occult master Tao Hongjing: *Recipes from Behind the Elbow for Every Emergency* (*Zhouhou beiji fang* 肘後備急方). Quotes of earlier lost texts are preserved in it as well as curious facts such as the earliest mention of smallpox (*tianhuabing* 天花病). Ge Hong is also credited with preserving a work by Hua Tuo called the *Golden Chest and the Green-Blue Satchel* (*Jinkui Lunang* 金匱綠囊). But this had also been lost until it was reinvented during the Song era, with names such as *Golden Chest Formulary* (*Jinkui fang* 金匱方) and *Jade Case Formulary* (*Yuhan fang* 玉函方), and attributed to Zhang Ji, the Han physician known for cold damage theory (Hanson, 2020, 81–82).

Materia medica, Magic, and Other Methods

Pharmaceutical literature was consolidated in the late medieval era throughout the Yuan era (1271–1368) and into early premodern times, incorporating ideas and *materia medica* from Inner Asia, South Asia, and the Middle East (Zheng et al., 2018, 13–18; Buell & Anderson, 2021, chap. 3). Some genuine early works (in contrast to forgeries of lost works) include one by the Tang official Wang Tao 王濤 (ca. 670–755). His *Arcane Essential Recipes from the Outer Censorate* (*Waitai miyao* 外臺秘要) incorporates discussions on the use of more than 6,000 recipes drawn from Tang and pre-Tang works. The first government-sponsored *materia medica*, called the *Newly Revised Materia Medica* (*Xinxiu bencao* 新修本草), produced by a team of Tang officials in 659, was based on Tao Hongjing's fifth-century work the *Collected Annotations on the Classic of Materia Medica* (*Bencao jing jizhu* 本草經記注) but was revised and updated with information collected from local regions in the Tang empire (Bian, 2020, 6–9; Liu, 2021, 30–1, 81–82, 92–94). Through these and other works, the use of many drugs still used in East Asian medicine today, such as aconite, can be traced back to the Han.

The importance of prayer, repentance, and timely behavior in Daoist healing is seen in the transmitted *Scripture on Great Peace* (*Taipingjing* 太平經). In response to epidemics in 171 CE, the leader of the Yellow Turban movement, Zhang Jue 張角, led followers to "confess their mistakes" before he administered talismans dissolved in water to them along with incantations

(Hendrischke, 2006, 19). Epidemics were believed to be caused by extravagant behavior or bad environmental *qi* (Hendrischke, 2006, 129, 144). Individual illnesses according to the *Scripture* could also be caused by people improperly "injuring the earth" (Hendrischke, 2006, 264). This concept is reflected in later geomancy practices and diagrams preserved in medieval manuscripts discovered in the northwestern desert cave complex of Dunhuang 敦煌 (Gansu). Some identify where the Earth Lord is residing on different days of the sexagenary calendar. This suggests that the body of the earth was viewed like the human body as being inhabited by different souls in different places at different times (Harper, 2005; Despeux, 2007). Not knowing the calendar could cause injury, illness, or even death if one performed acupuncture or dug a well at the wrong time or place.

General treatment approaches (not including the specificity of recipes) were consolidated by Chao Yuanfang 巢元方 (581–618) and others into the canon *Discourse on the Origins of Disease* (*Bingyuan lun* 病原論), also known as the *Discourse on the Origins and Symptoms of All Diseases* (*Zhubing yuanhou lun* 諸病源候論) (Zheng et al., 2018, 50). In 57 chapters, 1,739 disorders (*bing*) are named and discussed. In a late Qing edition (*Zhou shi yixue congshu* 周氏醫學 叢書, vol. 27), the illnesses are grouped into larger sections labeled as types of symptoms (*bing zhuhou*): "waist and back" (*yaobei* 腰背), "melting with thirst" (a symptom of diabetes) (*xiaoxie* 消瀉), "epidemics" (*yili* 疫癘), "all types of dripping" (*zhulin* 諸淋), and "moisture" (*shi* 濕) (Zhang & Unschuld, 2015, 567, 628, 692, 444). By far, the majority of ailments are classified as "moisture" syndromes. Dolly Yang has described the organization of the specific disorders as progressing from what was deemed most prevalent (such as "wind" or "deficiency" disorders), followed by disorders associated with meteorological factors, to those of the internal organs, parts of the head, visible injuries, and finally to specific disorders of women and children (Yang, 2018, 281–284).

Chao Yuanfang's canon frequently quotes from a lost text called *Nurturing Life Recipes* (*Yangsheng fang* 養生方), especially a chapter called "Guiding and Pulling Methods" ("Daoyin fa" 導引法), which may be linked in tradition to therapeutic exercise manuals discovered in Han tombs in Hunan and Hubei among manuscripts, including the self-titled *Pulling Book* (*Yinshu* 引書) from ZJS, about recipes, vessels, sex, and other topics (Harper, 1998, 110–119; Lo, 2014; Yang, 2018). The *Bingyuan lun* was first printed in the eleventh century from circulating manuscripts, and subsequent printed editions had an enormous impact on subsequent medical texts, including those of Japan and Korea (Yang, 2018, 263–269). This shows how difficult it is to determine the origin or date of a particular methodology and also how aspects of ancient practice persisted.

Chao Yuanfang's work no doubt influenced the Buddhist practitioner Sun Simiao's 孫思邈 (d. 682) encyclopedic canons of emergency medicine, *Essential Recipes for Emergencies Worth a Thousand Pieces of Gold* (*Beiji qianjin yaofang* 備急千金要方) and *Supplement to the Recipes Worth a Thousand Pieces of Gold* (*Qianjin yifang* 千金翼方). These included recipes as well as medical theory and discussions and treatments in the fields of pediatrics, gynecology, "seven openings" (of the body where external *qi* could penetrate) (*qiqiao* 七竅), wind ailments, "foot *qi*" (various ailments, some identified as beriberi) (*jiaoqi* 腳氣), cold damage, viscera, abscesses, "releasing toxins" (as required for fevers) (*jiedu* 解毒), dietetics, pulse-reading, and acumoxa. With more than 5,300 entries under 232 headings in 30 folios (*juan*), it is a massive text that is still being explored by modern scholars (Furth, 1999; Unschuld, 2000, 88–95; Engelhardt, 2001; Smith, 2008; Wilms, 2013, 2015; Sivin, 2017; Liu, 2021). We can find evidence of alchemy, spells, and hemerology as well as Daoist and Buddhist ideology mixed with more pragmatic medical approaches (Sivin, 2017; Lo, 2018, 592).

Early Chinese medical writings, including many no longer preserved in China, influenced the rise of medicine in Korea and Japan. Most notable is the collection of early texts preserved in the *Ishimpō* 醫心方 (*Remedies at the Heart of Medicine*) by Tanba no Yasuyori 丹波康賴 (ca. 912–95). Comparison of theories, terminology, and illustrations in the seventy-four medical manuscripts discovered among thousands of other scriptures, manuscripts, codices, and records hidden in Dunhuang help to date the ancient materials in the *Ishimpō*. Together, the *Ishimpō* and Dunhuang texts likewise provide a seventh-century date for a block-printed Chinese acumoxa text preserved only in Japan, the *Huangdi hamajing* 皇帝蛤蟆經 (*Toad Canon of Huangdi*) (Lo, 2001). Some of the evidence includes illustrations of acumoxa points on naked or near-naked men, numbers and names of points that vary from those in the canons, and, most significantly, the theory that five different kinds of spirit rotated inside the body, occupying different sites according to the calendar and the age of the person – thus setting up prohibition standards for where on the body one could needle without causing harm. This practice can be traced back to an Eastern Han medical manuscript from a tomb in Hantanpo 旱灘坡, Wuwei 武威, Gansu.

3 Non-transmitted Texts: From the Twelfth Century BCE to the Eleventh Century CE

Texts written on bone, bamboo, silk, and paper preserve versions of original documents that were buried and lost to time and thus were not subject to later revision. Before the era of court-sponsored textual production and preservation in the Han, medical information was embedded in technical and divination texts concerning a large array of personal or political topics. During the early imperial era, language concerning "ailments" (*bing*) began to be separated out from other topics. The mixed texts produced before then preserve ancient thought processes concerning illness and healing, much of which never made it into later canons and persisted in popular practice.

Pre-Han non-transmitted materials include divination records and manuals as well as narrative documents that are historical or philosophical in type. The earliest texts are divination records. Two sets of divination records are preserved: late Shang writing (twelfth-century BCE), most especially on turtle plastrons, and late Zhou bamboo records (fourth-century BCE). The Shang bones reflected the political and personal issues of the royal family and the fourth-century-BCE texts reflected the personal issues of politically connected elite men and their families. Generally, the primary mode of healing documented was exorcism and sacrifice directed at supernatural agencies, including human and nature spirits. Illness was understood as a symptom of "malign influence, catastrophe, curse" (*sui* 祟).

Shang Bone Inscriptions: Ancestral Powers

The diviners that accompanied the late Shang kings around the metropolis that would later be named Yinxu 殷墟 (Anyang, Henan) used a range of animal bones to divine, most commonly the water buffalo scapula. By the time of King Wu Ding 武丁 (ca. 1254 BCE–1197 BCE), however, the use of turtle plastrons reflected prestige and perhaps a supernatural connection to the Four Quadrate (*sifang* 四方) Shang cosmos (Allan, 1991, 101, 106–107, 111–113, 121). Records of diviners negotiating with the ancestors on how to heal "affliction" (*ji* 疾) in the bodies of the king and his family, especially those of his wives and his sons (various *zi* 子), are inscribed on turtle plastrons. The oracle bone inscriptions (hereafter OBI) record afflictions in the body (*shen* 身) or in a body part, such as the bones, head, eyes, nose, ears, mouth, teeth, tongue, the neck or throat, the upper arms, elbows, abdomen, thighs or crotch, buttocks, legs, and possibly the knees, feet, and toes (there is some debate on how to decipher some of these terms; Hu Houxuan, 1942; Fan Yuzhou, 1998; Du Zhengsheng, 2005, 83–88; Huang Tianshu, 2006, 151, 356–357). These all represent the outer visible body. There are a few cases that mention "heart" (*xin* 心), which in late Zhou records could refer either to the upper front torso of the outer body or to the inner self and source of emotion.

The diviners proposed questions (positive and negative alternatives) regarding the affliction. One question asked was to determine if "there is toxin" (*you du* 有蛊 > 毒) or not. The questions were directed through the OBI to the ancestors, who were considered either the source of the affliction and/or an agent for protection and healing (Tsung-tung Chang, 1970, 34–45; Cook, in press). To deflect negative ancestral power, exorcism or a warding-off ritual (*yu* 禦) was performed (Keightley, 2012, 356). Sacrifices were provided to persuade ancestral action. Critical to the performance was the choice of day and the number and types of animals to sacrifice. Answers to the questions were interpreted from the sounds and cracks the bones displayed when hot pokers were pressed into particular sites on the bones. These bones had been specially prepared with regular patterns of scraped notches on the back that connected to the points chosen to scorch on the front, suggesting a purposeful awareness of the bone, which, like the human body, was composed of a front and back that are connected by sensation or pain. Scholars suggest that the process linked, at least theoretically, to later cauterization or acumoxa practices (Hu Houxuan, 1984, 27–30; Harper, 1998, 96; Lewis, 2006b, 56, 72).

Just as later divination texts discussed medical issues in the context of other life concerns, the OBI embedded questions about the physical bodies of the king and his household with other concerns according to the sexagenary ritual calendar. The concept of "affliction" was not limited to the human body but could also be suffered by the social political body if, for example, outsiders invaded the Shang territory. We can envisage that, as Sivin noted for the individual medical body in early imperial times, the imagined king's body extended beyond his physical self (Sivin, 1995; Lloyd & Sivin, 2002, 214–226). Through the medium or proxy of the Four Quadrate–shaped plastron (representing the cosmos), diviners could diagnose issues within the larger social, political, and cosmic bodies of the king (Hanson, 2020). These OBI bones were specially prepared, a duty supervised by royal women. Once the bones were used, they were collected in a cache and buried. The conception of the bone as body and its burial in a mass grave is suggestive of its social agency as a body-servant to the king.

The relationship of the Four Quadrate–shaped plastron to the king's personal and extended body is difficult to untangle. One reason is the fragmented nature of the oracle bone evidence. But recently a cache of hundreds of relatively complete plastrons belonging to Wu Ding's sons was found in the eastern section of Huayuanzhuang 花園莊 burial ground: they provide clues (Huang Tianshu, 2006). An analysis of all the bones that mention "affliction" reveal first and foremost the primacy of time as an influential factor. The royal ancestral spirits were named according to the ten-day system, with male spirits occupying the beginning of the cycle and females (and possibly deceased elder brothers) at the end. There was definitely a correlation between the name of the day chosen for a sacrifice and that of the ancestor named to receive it. Over the course of a ritual period that a single plastron was used, different sections of the bone were used on different days in patterns on both its front and back, along the edges, and in the center spaces. The diviners were extremely conscious of symmetry, suggesting an early attention to the balance of supernatural forces within the proxy body of the turtle.

One challenge with all newly discovered archaic texts is deciphering the meaning of many archaic graphs. For the oracle bones, the logographic nature of the graphs can sometimes provide hints to the larger concepts behind a word's meaning if the word has no descendant graph or word that appears in transmitted text. For example, the toxic state caused by an external supernatural agency was written as 𝕚, a graph composed of a "foot" 止 on top of a "snake, worm, centipede, creature, bug" 虫. The word is understood as having no descendant graph and is read as a generalized "harm" (*hai* 害, Takashima, 2010, vol. 2, 150–153). In fact, it may represent an unrecognized variant for "toxic, poison" (*du* 毒) (Liu, 2021, 22; Cook, in press). This "bug" imagery appears in later paleographic contexts as a representation of outside supernatural influences; in medieval Daoist lore, bugs inside the body cause decay and death (Harper, 1998, 74–75; Strickmann, 2002, 36–37, 77–78; Unschuld, 2003, 180–189; Harper & Kalinowski, 2017, 129–133).

An ailment called *gu* 蠱 is depicted by a graph with bugs or creatures inside a vessel to represent a kind of toxic potion but also a bodily affliction. In the Shang, it seems to be linked to bone and teeth pain; in later texts, it was associated with sexual behavior and intestinal parasites (Cook, 2016). While it was mostly identified as afflicting a single body, there is one OBI in which it afflicted an entire non-Shang people; a suggested cure was extermination of the people. This radical solution suggests a fear of contagion. In the MWD manuscripts, it was considered a demonic ailment. Various treatments are noted: (1) ingesting the burnt dust of a bat or of a menstrual cloth; (2) applying a tincture with charred rooster comb and snake; (3) applying a tincture with menstrual blood mixed with cinnamon (Harper, 1998, 151, 300–302). In medieval times, *gu* was not just the name of an affliction; it was itself a demonic power, one that could cause chronic or acute illnesses and that must be expunged with strong drugs, such as realgar, croton, aconite, or centipede (Liu, 2021, 71–72).

Another descriptive ancient graph is the one for "affliction," written in a variety of ways such as with a body on a planchette with a hand over it holding some sort of implement 𝕚, a body on a planchette surrounded by drops of liquid 𝕚, or by many hands 𝕚. The reclined body on the bed or table-like structure suggests the patient; the hand holding an implement, or the hovering drops and multiple hands, may suggest treatment methods. Interestingly, the variant graphs for a Zhou term for the vanquished Shang people, *yin* 殷, was written as 𠂤𠂤, which in the rare OBI usage possibly refers to a medical technique. This graph also shows a hand with an implement over a body. The ancient graph for "body" (*shen*) also has many variants, some depicting an infant inside the rounded abdomen, suggesting that the graph represented both embodiment and reproduction (Cook & Luo, 2017, 95–96). Instruments mentioned in Han texts include lancing stones, hammers, sticks, reeds, and arrows (Harper, 1998, 161, 169). An oracle bone graph possibly of "bug" and a "hand holding something" (possibly the latter rare word meaning "to spread" 攽 or 攱), used in the sense of "to dismember" (a human sacrificial victim) (Chen Guangyu et al., 2017, 189–190). The Shang people may have practiced a procedure, either exorcist or surgical, that the Zhou found barbaric and thus used as a disparaging reference for a vanquished people.

An ancient form of healing, involving binding the evil spirit, may be implied in this undeciphered OBI graph 𠂤. It depicts two hands holding a knotted cord and may link to later exorcistic healing methods using knotted bound forms, twisted body postures, or other actions described by Donald Harper interpreting a third-century-BCE text called "spellbinding, accusing" (*jie* 詰) (Harper, 1985, 475–476). Binding harmful presences could involve oral pronouncements (*gao* 告), evident in both OBI and later texts that employ magical medicine. The OBI graph for "to ward off, exorcise" (*yu*) depicts a kneeling person with a knotted cord 𦐇 (simplified to 𦐇). Healing *sui* (malign supernatural influence) involving exorcism would persist for thousands of years, although the particular undeciphered OBI graph seems to have disappeared.

Like ancient graphs, material culture preserves a few hints. The appearance of tiny jade and bone knives and a variety of vessels and implements preserved in tombs may imply a role for superficial surgeries and herbal decoctions. However, unlike Qin and Han bamboo and silk texts, OBI only document exorcism and sacrifice rituals to counter the effect of external influences, natural and man-made, on the king's social and personal body (Allan, 1991; Keightley, 2000). We see the predominance of the royal body as subject until the fourth century BCE materials reveal a shift to concern with the individual bodies of elite males.

Zhou Bronze Inscriptions and Bamboo Manuscripts: The Rise of *Qi*

From the mid-eleventh to the mid-third century BCE, the literate population expanded beyond the royal court into myriad regions along the Yellow and Yangzi river valleys. Regional diversity continued to increase due to trade, war, and migration. Three types of texts preserve Zhou-era writing: bronze inscriptions, bamboo manuscripts, and transmitted texts. Bamboo texts are the most revealing of the three because they tend to be records buried with specific individuals. Some tales reflecting medical ideology are also found in bamboo books or in transmitted chronicles. The bronze inscriptions date from the late Shang up to the end of the Zhou; the bamboo manuscripts are from the fifth century BCE up through the Qin and Han periods; the relevant transmitted texts are believed to date from roughly the sixth to the third century BCE. We see a persistent use of magical medicine in these texts but a shift in concepts of the body and evidence of new concepts, such as *qi*.

Bronze inscriptions memorialize court rituals and the relationship of individuals to the king. Individuals' bodies are mentioned as extensions of their king's physical being. Parts of the body – the "heart" (*xin*), "abdomen-and-heart" (*fuxin* 腹心), and "(upper) arms and (upper) legs, limbs" (*gongu* 肱股) – are terms used to explain the extent of the individual's loyalty and dedication to the king's mission. They were expected "to exhaust" (*jin* 盡) their bodies while also "modeling" (*xing* 型) ancestral patterns of loyalty to their kings. In reward, their hearts (representing their inner selves) would be filled with "bright, luminous" (*ming* 明) "potency, virtue" (*de* 德) (Cook, 2017; Ke Heli, 2022). In later times, after the eighth century BCE, when the Zhou kings were chased out of their homeland by the Rong people and lost their legitimacy and connection to Heaven (the ultimate source of the power *de*), individuals tried to draw down *de* or *yang qi* directly from Heaven. By the fourth century BCE, the ruler was a symbol internalized in the body of the educated elite man (the *junzi* 君子); he was the "heart" or "center, inner" (*zhong* 中) and the limbs symbolized his ministers (Chen Wei, in press). Later, in Han transmitted texts, the ministers were the inner "depots" of *qi* (viscera) with channels or *mai* as circuits of communication between them and their ruler, the heart.

The earliest graphic form of the word *qi* appears in fourth-century BCE bamboo strips preserved in Chu tombs, despite a transmitted textual tradition linking it to court-sponsored debates in the northeast (Harper, 1999a, 824–825; Needham, 2000, 43). Recent scholarship shows that the Han graph for *qi*, written with "cloud" or "vapor" 气 over "grain" 米, was likely due to the Qin tendency to confuse *qi* with the word for *xi* 餼 *qʰ(r)ə[t]-s, "a gift of food." Chu bamboo texts write it with a phonetic *[k]ə[t]-s 既 over one of two semantic signifiers, representing either "fire" 火 or "heart" 心 (Cook, 2021; phonetic reconstructions from Baxter & Sagart, 2014; see also Lo & Stanley-Baker, 2022, 23–50). In later cosmic medicine, Fire is the element or Agency linked to the "heart."

Bamboo and silk philosophical texts from the fourth century BCE provide clues to the nature of *qi*. Aging and growth are processes of *qi*, with the peak being during the stage of sexual maturity (*zhuang* 壯); females are distinguished as having more *yin qi* and males with more *yang qi* (Cao, 2019, 116–117, 120–125;

Cook, 2019, 187–190; Guo, 2019, 225–23; Huang, 2019). Hot and cold *qi* was linked to geography and "blood" (*xue*) to kinship and to those parts of the body not defined by muscle and skin (Jingmenshi bowuguan, 1998, *Liu de* 六德 strip 15, *Tang Yu zhi dao* 唐虞之道 strip 11). Blood and *qi* were controlled by the heart (Hsu, 2008–9). Self-cultivation practices or "Techniques of the Heart" (*xinshu* 心術) allowed one to moderate affective types of *qi* (Jingmenshi bowuguan, 1998, *Laozi* 老子A strip 35; *Xing zi ming chu* 性自命出 strips 2 and 44). This involved "rectifying" (*zheng* 正) the human "intention, will" (*zhi* 志) for an individual's inner harmony, or even for the pacification of an entire people. *Qi* also represented the productive aspects of Heaven and Earth (*tiandi*) and *yinyang* (Ma Chengyuan, 2001–12, Vol. 2, *Min zhi fumu* 民之父母 strips 12–13, *Rongchengshi* 容成氏 strips 29–30; Jingmenshi bowuguan, 1998, *Taiyi sheng shui* 太一生水 strip 10).

The concept of "primordial *qi*" (*yuanqi* 元氣), something beyond life and death and thus a key to immortality, is understood as a Han idea. But in the fourth-century-BCE bamboo manuscript called the *Hengxian* 恆先, there is the term "eternal *qi*" (*heng qi* 恆氣), which formed the central balancing mechanism or "pole, pivot" (*ji* 極) of the cosmos. It was self-generating and could split into clear and turbid forms that condensed into Heaven and Earth (Ma Chengyuan, 2001–12, Vol. 3, strips 1, 2, 4, 9). Understanding the nature of *qi* was one step toward enlightenment, although unlike the late Han and early medieval ideas of bodily escape, it was seen as a tool for leadership (Brindley, 2013; Cook, 2013a; Perkins, 2013).

The application of the concept of *qi* in a medical context appears first in the fourth-century-BCE bamboo divination and sacrifice manuscript discovered in a Chu tomb in Baoshan 包山, Hubei. This records three years of attempts by a team of diviners, who specialized in ten different methods, used in rotation, to diagnose the afflictions of an ailing member of the Chu elite. While they focused on identifying the demonic agent that caused the ailment, the symptoms included *qi* flowing in reverse (*ni* 逆) or "up" (*shang* 上), which resulted in an afflicted "heart" (*xin*) or "heart-and-abdomen" (*xinfu*) (the upper and lower front body). Weakness or shallow breath was "scarce" (*shao* 少) *qi* (Cook, 2006; Ke Heli, 2021). The movement of *qi* either up or down reflects a much simpler model of inner circuitry than imagined in the *HDNJ* and later canons. The MWD *Model of the Vessels* (*Maifa*) of the second century BCE explains it as follows (Ma Jixing, 1992, 247–282; Harper, 1998, 213):

> The model of the vessels [should be] clarified for the lower [people] as it was valued by the sages. As for *qi*, it benefits the lower part [of the body] and harms the upper part as it follows warmth and goes away from coolness to it (lower part). This is why sages have cold heads and warm feet. To heal ailments, remove surplus [*qi*] and supplement what is lacking.

以脈法明教下脈亦聖人所貴也。氣也者利下而害上從暖而去清焉。
故聖人寒頭而暖足。治病者取有餘而益不足也。

In fourth-century-BCE bamboo manuscripts, the body is spatially divvied up in two ways: front-and-back and inner-and-outer. Similar but more fragmented records than those from Baoshan have been discovered in other tombs inhabited by Chu officials: in Wangshan 望山 and Tianxingguan 天星觀 in Hubei and in Xincai 新蔡 (also referred to as Geling 葛陵 by some scholars) in Henan. Chu records refer to the trunk of the body as "heart" (*xin*), "back" (*bei* 背), "abdomen-and-heart" (*fuxin* or *xinfu*), and as "back-and-chest" (*beiying* 膺), or "chest and ribs" (*xiongxie* 胸脅). Only the "abdomen-and-heart" suffered afflictions of breath or appetite, suggesting some sense of internal function, confirming Elisabeth Hsu's idea that *qi* represented the invisible inner aspect of the outer visible form (*xing* 形) (Hsu, 2008–9). The trunk (including front-and-back) could suffer from "bloating" (*pangzhang* 胖脹). Besides *qi*, another aspect of the inner body mentioned is bones. An affliction in the foot (or lower leg) bones is mentioned in the Wangshan record and the entire skeleton, the "one-hundred bone body" (*baiguti* 百骨體), is mentioned in the Xincai record. The most common locution for "body" found in all the fourth-century-BCE records is *gongshen* 躬身 (Cook, 2006; Ke Heli, 2021); Deborah Sommer (2008) notes that, in transmitted texts, *ti* implied bodies formed out of component parts, whereas *gong* indicated separate individuals.

While front-and-back were clearly concepts since the Shang OBI, the evolving senses of inner-and-outer are evident in fourth-century-BCE bamboo manuscripts. The *Stalk Divination* (*Shifa* 筮法) (hereafter *Stalk*) manuscript, as it is titled by Tsinghua University scholars, likely came from the same region as the Baoshan manuscript. In this divination manual (about the size of a placemat and easily rolled for carrying), a drawing of the human body is included in a chart for easy reference. It was drawn facing forward placed within a cosmograph of influencing cosmic agencies including direction, season, and time. *Yin* and *yang* are not stated; only four of the Five Agents are mentioned, suggesting that the fifth and missing Agent – Earth – later representing the Center and the emperor, and the *wuxing* system, was a product of the early imperial age.

Another pre-imperial aspect is the focus on male and female agencies representing cosmic forces such as the phases of the moon and the seasons. They were symbolized in the manuscript by eight stacks of three numbers derived from stalk or dice divination. These named trigrams are familiar as the building blocks of the sixty-four hexagrams in the *Book of Changes* (*Yijing* 易經), a popular Han philosophical text derived from a Zhou divination manual (the *Zhouyi*) and used in late medieval medical diagnosis. But the earlier manuscript had no philosophical dimension. It was a pragmatic method for diagnosing problems. Trigram patterns were interpreted to determine, for example, if someone would live or die. The trigrams also were responsible for different sites on the body. The outer rim of the body is marked with male trigrams: top of the head, ears, hands, and feet. The inner sections of the body are marked with female trigrams: face, upper chest (heart), lower chest (abdomen), and inside the upper thighs. The most powerful trigrams (Qian 乾 and Kun 坤), the ones composed of pure male and female numbers, mark the top of the head and the heart respectively. The eight trigrams, which marked sections of the body, also correlated to lists of ghosts and demons that might be sources of *sui* (Cook & Zhao, 2017, 131–139).

The inner-and-outer distinction is also reflected in the comparisons of symptoms listed in divination records recovered from Chu burials in Hubei and Henan. The troubles of the deceased, of Shao Tuo 邵佗, a minister (*zuoyin* 左尹), in the Baoshan record and of Shao Gu 邵固 in the Wangshan record, were both described as "heart" conditions with restricted bodily movement. Shao Tuo suffered from reverse and scarce *qi*. Shao Gu suffered from blockage or congestion (*yi sai* 以塞) and diarrhea (*shanbian* 善便) (strips 17–18; Chen Wei, 2009, 272, 279). In Wangshan strip 38, this condition is further described as a "contracted bowel" (*ju bian* 聚便, read by some as an "urgent bowel," *zhoubian* 驟便) and curiously listed together with an affliction of the foot bones (*zugu ji* 足骨疾) (Cook, 2006, 261; Chen Wei, 2009, 272, 280). A perceived connection between functions of the heart, abdomen, and legs hints at the route of a foot vessel as described in the later MWD manuscripts, suggesting perhaps a rudimentary conception of a *mai* system.

Shao Wang 邵王, Lord of Pingye 坪夜君, of the Xincai record was afflicted with bloating and a heart condition (strips A3, 219, 117, 120; Chen Wei, 2009, 405, 435). Fansheng, Lord of Diyang 邸陽君番勝, whose suffering is recorded in the Tianxingguan record, suffered from the same back, chest, and heart ailments but also chills ("cold and hot," *cangran* 滄然) and grief (*qiqi* 戚戚 for 慼慼), which caused a suppression of his appetite, aggravated by a dry throat (*yi gan* 嗌幹) (Yan Changgui, 2004, 276–277). The psychological aspect of illness persists as a diagnosable symptom throughout Qin and Han manuscripts and points to the role of "heart" as both a physical location and a source of invisible *qi*.

Shao Tuo of Baoshan suffered "anxiety, troubles" (*you* 憂). Some scholars read the *you* as *qi* 慼 ("distress"), a synonym attested in Han dictionaries. The condition of *qiqi* was linked in the *Analects* (論語 *Lunyu*) to something suffered by "lesser people" (*xiaoren* 小人) ("Shu er" 述而 37). In a Han tale of a medical case attributed to the legendary Bian Que, a patient is described as *qiqi*. This young woman was experiencing chills and was near death. He felt her pulse and pronounced "worm conglomeration" (*raoxia* 蟯瘕) (Hsu, 2010, 84). The *Records of History* (*Shiji* 史記) explain that "the ailment of *raoxia* involves abdominal bloating and yellowed and coarse skin, and when stroking [the pulse] [feels] like a condition of *qiqi*" (蟯瘕為病, 腹大, 上膚黃麤, 循之戚戚然). Commentaries note that this condition of *qiqi* involves feeling of "movement" (*dong* 動) in the heart – a Han description of pathological agitation felt in a vessel (Hsu, 2010, 84–85). In the fourth-century-BCE Guodian 郭店 bamboo strips, the condition of *qi* 戚 (read as *qi* 慼) is said to derive from "anxiety" (*you*), resulting from excessive "movement" (*dong*) of the heart, also known as "congested emotion" (*yun* 慍 "anger"). Interestingly, the original graph written for "congested emotion" was 囚 ("prisoner") over a heart 心, which might also be translated as *qiu* 怬, "brooding," although scholars prefer to read it as *yun* (Jingmenshi, *Xing zi ming qu* 性自命出, strip 34; Chen Wei, 2009, 222). Han recipes for "heart blockage" (*xinbi* 心痹) continue to include a similar psychological dimension.

A word used to describe a heart condition that appears in the records of Wangshan, Tianxingguan, and Xincai (but not Baoshan) is read as *mian* or *men* 悗 ("heart pressure, confused"), defined as "gloomy, grieved" (*men* 懣, 悶) (Hubeisheng wenwu kaogu yanjiusuo et al, 1999, 146–147; Yan Changgui, 2004, 276; Chen Wei, 2009, 279 n. 13). This heart condition occurs in the context of symptoms causing "anxiety, trouble" (*you* or *qi*) for which the diviners were charged to find the source (*gu* 故) of the curse (*sui*) and then "attack" (*gong* 攻) it (a magical procedure). The examples that follow are selected from longer divinatory statements (Chen Wei, 2009; Liu Xinfang, 2011):

Baoshan Strip 207: 病腹疾以少氣

The ailment is an affliction in the abdomen, with a scarcity of *qi*

Strips 218, 220: 以其下心而疾少氣

With it going below the heart and afflicting (Shao Tuo) with scarcity of *qi*

Strips 221, 223: 既有病病心疾少氣不內食

[He] already has an ailment which is a heart affliction, with scarcity of *qi* and loss of appetite

Strips 236, 239, 242, 245, 248: 既腹心疾以上氣不甘食

[He] already is afflicted in the abdomen-and-heart with rising *qi* and loss of appetite

Wangshan 1 Strip 9: 既痤以悗心不內食

Already [has] swellings (boils?), with heart pressure and no appetite

Strip 13: 既痤以心悗 (?) 然不可以動 (?) 思遷身痿(?)

Already [has] swellings, with heart pressure, inability to think clearly or move his body, weakness

Strip 17: 既心悗以塞善弁 (便?) [broken]

   Already [has] heart pressure with obstructions and much easing of the bowels

Strip 37: [broken] 不能食以心悗以弁胸臘 (脅) 疾 [broken]

   Cannot eat, with heart pressure, and with easing of the bowels and affliction in the chest and ribs

Strip 38: [broken] 以心悗不能食以聚 (驟) 弁足骨疾 [broken]

   With heart pressure and inability to eat, with urgent easing of the bowels and affliction in the foot bones

Xincai A1 Strip 14: 背膺疾以胅脹心悗 [broken]

   Affliction in the back-and-chest, with bloating and heart pressure

A3 Strip 100 既背膺疾以胛以心 [broken]

   Already is afflicted in the back-and-chest, with [problems] in the shoulders and the heart

A3 Strip 189 既心悗胅脹以百骨體疾

   Already has heart pressure, bloating, with affliction in the skeleton.

A3 Strip 233 既心疾以會於背且心悗 [broken]

   Already afflicted in the heart, with convergence [of bad *qi*?] in the back and then [causing] heart pressure

Note that each patient shares the same contingent symptoms. While all share heart pressure, some suffer from lack of appetite, others from chest or back pain, or from diarrhea. Shao Tuo of Baoshan had problems with his *qi* moving up and down between his heart and abdomen, with the final reversal causing the diviner to ask if it would cause him to die (*shang wu si* 尚毋死). In bamboo strips from a Qin tomb in Zhoujiatai 周家台, Hubei (dated to around 213 BCE–210 BCE), a similar heart affliction is defined as a *jia* 瘕 syndrome, "congestion, conglomeration," in which the normal flow of *qi* and perhaps other bodily elements, such as blood or "essence, spirit" (*jing*), is blocked. In the second-century-BCE Han text from LGS, known as the *Liushi bingfang* 六十病方 (strips 494, 532, 626), "successive congestion" (*chengjia* 承瘕) is described as fatal when it moves up and down within the heart-and-abdomen, resulting in bloating in the rib area and trembling and breaking out in sweat. Similar symptoms are described for "chest congestion" (*xiong jia* 胸瘕) in another LGS text, the *Zhubing* 諸病 2 (strip 415). In this case, the patient feels equal pain in the back and chest. The text specifically categorizes this illness as "heart blockage" (*xin bi* 心痹) (Hubeisheng Jingzhoushi Zhouliang yuqiao yizhi bowuguan, 2001, 131; Lin Zhenbang, 2019, 141; Wang Yitong, 2019, 3–6).

   The heart condition *mian* 悗 is explained as "heart pressure" in the *HDNJ Lingshu* and as caused by overindulgence in sweet foods. Huangdi asks about the situation of sweetness coursing through the flesh of the body and why it results in *mian*. The minister Shao Yu explains that sweet flavors that enter the stomach are a weak type of *qi* incapable of rising to the Upper Burner (upper third of the trunk) and thus lingering in the stomach, setting up a moist soft environment for "bugs" to thrive. The bugs cause heart pressure and then the *qi* of sweetness goes into the flesh (黃帝曰: 甘走肉, 多食之. 令人悗心, 何也? 少俞曰: 甘入于胃, 其氣弱小, 不能上至於上焦, 而與谷留於胃中者, 令人柔潤者也, 胃柔則緩, 緩則蟲動, 蟲動則令人悗心. 其氣外通於肉, 故甘走肉) (Unschuld, 2016a, 574–575). Elsewhere in the *Lingshu*, the problem of insufficient lower *qi* results in loss of physical mobility (*wei* 痿), receding *qi* (a condition known as *jue* 厥), and heart pressure (*xin mian*) (下氣不足, 則乃為痿厥心悗;) (Unschuld, 2016a, 337). This is one of a series of cases when "perverse *qi*" gets into the body. Elsewhere in the *Lingshu*, the problem of too much or too little *qi* is discussed. Too much results in the chest (*xiong*) feeling full with pressured breathing (*mian xi* 息); too little results in not even being able to talk (Unschuld, 2016a, 364). We see a clear transition to *yinyang wuxing* correlative medicine in the *HDNJ* versus the simpler explanations in the fourth-through second-century-BCE manuscripts.

Among the cases of Bian Que described in the *Shiji* is one about a case of an infant feeling "upset and oppressed" (*fan men* 煩懣) due to an ailment of blocked *qi* (氣鬲病; 病使人煩懣). Symptoms include inability to keep food or drink down caused by "anxiety" (*you*). Bian Que used a concoction to get the *qi* to properly descend and get the child eating again. He then worked on the heart *qi* to balance out the overly strong *yang* caused by the body being hot (身熱) and the food not being ingested, causing excessive (blood) in the vessels (絡脈有過). If the blood had risen, the patient would die. It was all caused by a "sad heart" (*bei xin* 悲心) (Hsu, 2010, 74–75). In the *HDNJ*, the term *fanmen* 煩悶 ("vexation") is linked to heart pain and *fanyuan* 煩寃 ("vexation and grievance") is connected to a feeling of fullness in the abdomen (Tessenow & Unschuld, 2008, 108). In Qin and Han manuscripts, *fan* suggests a serious stage of an illness. In a manner somewhat reminiscent of oracle bone piercing, "heart blockage" in the Han was treated with paired needling of the back-and-front (*HDNJ Lingshu* 7, "Guan zhen" 官鍼; Unschuld, 2016a, 141).

The etiology of congested or distressed hearts is reminiscent of fourth-century-BCE cases: excessive sad emotion, overindulgence in a particular taste, and invasion of a demonic influence. The symptoms also include bloating and scarcity of *qi*. The Han texts go further in their conception of what is occurring inside the body and use methods to interpret it – such as pulse-reading and interpreting facial complexions – and methods of healing – such as administering decoctions or acumoxa – that are not mentioned in late Zhou texts. For the late Zhou, the situation of affliction and healing through exorcism is explained by the philosopher Hanfeizi 韓非子: "The afflictions of people are caused by ghosts cursing" (鬼祟也疾人) but "ghosts harming people" (鬼傷人) is reversed by the "harm" people cause ghosts through exorcism rituals (人逐除之之謂人傷鬼也) ("Jie lao" 解老, Wang Xianshen, 1991, 104).

Diviners used specialized tools (turtles, stalks, and others) to identify afflicting spirits, any number of powerful human ancestors, anonymous ghosts, or the spirits of built spaces and of terrestrial and celestial forms. If the spirit could be named, it received sacrifices and prayers according to a hierarchical system of offerings including animal sacrifice and gifts of jade and clothing. Healers "willed and attacked [the ghost] to resolve [the affliction]" (*si gong jie* 思攻解) (Yan Changgui, 2004, 289–291). They used force of mind (their own heart *qi*?) as well as possibly implements to attack (*gong* 攻) or send off (*shi* 使) the spirit. The verb "willed" (*si* 思) sometimes alternated in the same rhetorical formula with the word "command" (*ming* 命), suggesting also the force of words. Harper (1998, 92–93) calls the "release" (*jie* 解) of the body from demonic possession an elimination ritual (see also Lo, 2002b; Cook, 2006, 84–85). In one MWD manuscript, the *Recipes for Fifty-Two Ailments* (*Wushier bingfang* 五十二病方) (hereafter *Recipes*), the healer first invoked the paired powers of Sun-and-Moon and Mother-and-Father, then verbally threatened the harmful spirits with an actual (or symbolic?) beating (*ji* 擊) using a hammering stone (*duan shi* 鍛石). Other words used for hammering demons include *gai* (毅, 敁) and *duan* 段. Instead of a stone, an iron mallet (*tie chui* 鐵椎) might be used (Ma Jixing, 1992, 477; Harper, 1998, 148, 261, sec. 120). A conceptual parallel can be drawn between the use of pointed implements to exorcise demons from the body in magical medicine and the rise of needling practices to control *qi* in cosmic medicine. The healing movements were the same even if the rationales had different names.

The late Zhou approach to illness and healing is revealed also in narrative tales about corrupt rulers whose physical bodies and territorial states suffer in tandem, showing a continuation of the ruler's social body but with an added moral component (Riegel, 2012–13; Caboara, 2016). In the transmitted versions of these tales, healing required behavioral modification instead of sacrifices, prayers, and exorcism, suggesting later editing in an attempt to move away from demonography. The bamboo manuscript versions still value addressing the spirits, but, notably, specific ailments are named instead of just listing symptoms or afflicted parts of the body as seen in the divination texts. The Shanghai Museum bamboo book collection preserves two such tales: *Jian Dawang bo han* 柬大王泊 (迫) 旱 (*The Great King Jian Suffers the Drought*) and *Jing Gong nüe* 競公瘧 (*Lord Jing's nüe-Fever*) (Ma Chengyuan, vols. 4 & 6).

In the first tale, the state was experiencing a drought, after the king had conquered new territory. The king, known in transmitted texts as King Jian of Chu 楚簡王 (r. 431 BCE–408 BCE), exposed himself to the sun in an ancient rain ritual and ended up with a debilitating skin condition, *jie* 疥 (itchy skin disorder, scabies), which over prolonged exposure could develop into *saoshu bing* 瘙(瘙)鼠(瘑)病 (itchy pustules ailment) (Zhang Qixian et al., 2014, 4; Ma Chengyuan, 2001–12, Vol. 4, 199). Therefore, the diviner in charge, Turtle Minister (*guiyin* 龜尹), suggested shortcuts to the proper rituals to the new territory's mountains and streams. But another officer warned that upsetting "the standards of the spirits" (*guishen zhi chang* 鬼神之常) would offend them. Dream analysis confirmed the identity of the primary offended spirit, Drought Mother (Hanmu 旱母), possibly another name for the demon Siba 槐魆, mentioned as a source of curses and associated with afflictions of the mouth in the *Stalk* (Cook & Zhao, 2017, 136). Once the king repaired the altars, performed the proper sacrifices, and treated the people benevolently, the sun no longer made him ill and the rain came.

The ruler, Lord Jing of Qi 齊景公 (r. 547 BCE–490 BCE), of the second tale also suffered from *jie* (the archaic graph was written with an added "bug" semantic) due to bad behavior (Riegel, 2012–13, 228–229; Caboara, 2016, 58). The transmitted versions specifically rejected the notion of ghosts and unhappy spirits, but the bamboo version blamed the king's severe feverish chills (*nüe* 瘧) on prolonged exposure to the wind (strip 2 recto) and to ineffective invocators and astrologists (*zhushi* 祝史) (Riegel, 2012–13, 229). The transmitted version focuses on how the sage minister Yanzi 晏子 advocated moral behavior instead of the useless bribing of spirits, whereas the bamboo version focuses on the nature of the illness (Cao Jianguo, 2020).

The *nüe*-type of fever is often translated as malaria, although as with the name of any ancient ailment we cannot be sure of its precise biomedical identity. In the *HDNJ Suwen* "Nüe lun" 瘧論, different types of seasonal *nüe* (also called *kainüe* 痎瘧) affect different parts of the body, depending on the hot or cold nature of the *qi*. Symptoms include back pain, shortness of breath, nausea, and "vexation and grievance" (Unschuld & Tessenow, 2011, vol. 1, 535–552). The seasonal nature of *jie* and *nüe* is emphasized in the transmitted ritual canon the *Zhouli* 周禮:

> The Physician for Afflictions (*jiyi* 疾醫) is in charge of taking care of the myriad peoples' illnesses. Every season there is a pestilence (*liji* 癘疾): in the spring there is the scalp disorder (*xiaoshouji* 痟首疾, *xiao* is unknown, maybe a graphic variant for 消 "wasting"); in summer there is the itchy *jie*-skin disorder (*yangjieji* 痒疥疾); in the fall there is the *nüe*-cold disorder; and in winter there is the coughing-up of *qi* disorder (*sou shangqiji* 嗽上氣疾).

The physicians were instructed to treat the patients with dietetic and herbal medicines according to the Five Agents, five sounds, and five colors, checking for changes in the apertures (*qiao* 竅, acumoxa points) linked to problems in the viscera (Ruan Yuan, 1983, *Zhouli zhushu* 5.29).

The most famous Zhou tales of ill rulers are preserved in transmitted literature, including collections of historical tales such as the *Zuozhuan* 左傳 and the *Guoyü* 國語, along with references in philosophical texts, such as the *Hanfeizi*. These accounts also depict a struggle between different healing approaches. In a tale dated to 581 BCE, Lord Jing of Jin 晉景公 (r. 589–581) was treated first by a shaman of Mulberry Fields (Sangtian *wu* 桑田巫) and then Physician Huan 醫緩 from Qin 秦. The symptoms include two nightmares:

(1) the Lord being chased by a large *li* 厲 (pestilence demon) with long loose hair that reached the ground; and
(2) two boy demons hiding deep in the space between his heart and diaphragm.

Both dreams were interpreted (the first by the shaman and the second by the physician) as fatal. The pestilence demon was associated with the ghosts of those killed unjustly. Physician Huan noted that the location of the two small demons on top of the *huang* 肓 (the region between the heart and diaphragm in later medicine) and beneath the *gao* 膏 (fat) rendered useless the usual remedies of "attack" (*gong*), "reach and penetrate" (*da* 達), or "herbal decoctions" (*yao* 藥) (Wai-yee Li 2007, 240–242; Cook, 2013b, 18–21; Brown, 2015, 32). "Reaching and penetrating" is vocabulary employed later in acumoxa therapy.

A second account concerns the attempts to heal a later Jin ruler, Lord Ping of Jin 晉平公 (r. 557 BCE–524 BCE). He suffered from "urine retention" (*long* 癃) and was treated by a legendary minister Zichan 子產 (d. 522 BCE), originally of Zheng 鄭, and a Physician He 醫和 of Qin (Riegel, 2012–13, 233–241; Hanmo Zhang, 2013; Brown, 2015, 21–40). In the *Hanfeizi*, the physical ailment and a three-year drought were both caused by the ruler's interest in licentious music (Wang Xianshen, 1991, 44–45). Music was understood to stimulate the heart and cause emotion (*qing*) to rise out of the person's inner purpose or "intention" (*zhi*), a kernel of humanity lodged in the heart that one had to properly nurture in order to succeed in life (Wai-yee Li, 2005, 135; Cook, 2017, 225–241). In the *HDNJ Lingshu*, the ailment *long* is classed as a "heat" ailment that can present like *gu* poisoning in a male, blocked menses in a woman, and for either sex with a feeling of "dissolution" or "detachment" (*jie* 解) in the lower back accompanying a loss of appetite (Unschuld, 2016a, 302). The diagnosis of *gu* poisoning, linked to indulgence in sex with women with taboo clan names and at inauspicious times of the day, appears also in late Zhou accounts of Lord Ping's illness (*Zuozhuan* for 541 BCE; Liu, 2021, 73–78).

When Lord Ping became ill, diviners determined that the curse (*sui*) was caused by obscure star and land spirits, the deified sons of legendary emperors whose native lands had been trampled and ancestral sacrifices interrupted by the Jin. Zichan first shifted the focus from nature spirits to issues of morality; then Physician He confirmed the cause was neither ghosts nor bad diet but a fatal "bedroom disorder like *gu*" (*shiji ru gu* 室疾如蠱) that caused "confusion" (*huo* 惑) and weakened will (*zhi*). To be healed, the ruler must align action to cosmic agencies and proper timing, explained as the six *qi* of Heaven (*yin*, *yang*, wind, rain, darkness, light) as organized by the four seasons and the five nodes (*jie* 節), the five flavors, five colors, and five sounds. Excess *yin* causes a cold illness; excess *yang* a heat illness; excess wind results in limb afflictions; excess rain results in an abdominal illness; excess darkness causes confusion; and excess light afflicts the heart (Brown, 2015, 27). This is obviously a later editor's cosmic medical overlay and supports Miranda Brown's (2015, 39) suggestion that the figure of Physician He is "a contrived rhetorical device."

The contrived nature of the diagnosis in the transmitted tale is exacerbated by the use of the *Book of Changes* to confirm the diagnosis, a practice undocumented in early non-transmitted texts. The interpretation relies on a poetic description of the images Mountain over Wind linked to the two trigrams that make up the Gu hexagram, according to the *Shuogua* 說卦 (*Explaining Mantic Images*), a text transmitted as a commentary to the *Changes* (see Xing Wen in Cook, 2013b, 20–21). Notably, this commentary is also the only place in the *Changes* where the word "ailment, illness" (*bing*) appears. Only later Han derivations of the *Changes*, such as in the *Jiaoshi Yilin* 焦氏易林, mention specific ailments.

The *Shuogua* focus on how the eight trigrams link to the body recalls the fourth-century-BCE *Stalk* bamboo manual mentioned earlier in this section. In the *Shuogua*, the order of paired trigrams is as a gendered hierarchy of couples (male to female, high to low): Qian 乾 – Kun 坤, Zhen 震 – Xun 巽, Kan 坎 – Li 離, Gen 艮 – Dui 兌. Table 1 follows the *Stalk* order; basically male trigrams and odd numbered days are *yang*; female and even numbers, *yin*. Both texts claim to represent the Way of Heaven (*tian zhi dao* 天之道), but the *Shuogua* reflects the *Changes* tradition of taking Kan and Li as Water and Fire, whereas they are the exact opposite in the *Stalk*. The Stem + Number (S#) and Branch + Number (B#) correlations are from charts written under the cosmogram in the *Stalk*.

Notably absent in the *Shuogua* is the sexually charged journey described in the *Stalk* of the pair Kun and Qian meeting to birth the moon over the course of a month (Cook & Zhao, 2017, 126–127). Perhaps this served as a guide to the

Table 1 Trigram correlations

Trigram	Stalk Divination	Shuogua
Qian	Top of head Northwest S1, S9	Head (*shou* 首) Northwest, Heaven, Metal, Cold, Dark Red
Kun	Heart or chest Southwest S2, S10	Abdomen (*fu* 腹) Earth, Black
Gen	Lower arms and hands Northeast S3, B5, B11	Lower arms and hands (*shou* 手) Northeast, Mountain Finger (*zhi* 指)
Dui	Mouth and face West, Metal, White Supervisor of Receiving, Sishou 司收 S4, B6, B12	Mouth and tongue (*koushe* 口舌) Autumn, Swamp
Kan	Ears, sides of head South, Fire, Red. Supervisor of Planting, Sishu 司樹 S5, B3, B9	Ears (*er* 耳) North, Water "With regard to its application to people, it represents increased anxiety, heart ailment, ear pain, the mantic sign of blood, and red" 其於人也為加憂為心病為耳痛為血卦為赤.

Table 1 (cont.)

Trigram	Stalk Divination	Shuogua
Li	Abdomen North, Water, Black Supervisor of Storing, Sizang 司藏 S6, B4, B10	Eyes (*mu* 目) South, Fire, Sun "With regard to its application to people, it represents the main abdomen and the mantic sign of dryness (*qian*)" 其於人也為大腹大腹為乾卦.
Zhen	Lower legs and feet East, Wood, Green Supervisor of Thunder, Silei 司雷 S7, B1, B7	Lower legs and feet (*zu* 足) East, Dragon, Thunder, Dark Yellow
Xun	Inner thighs and crotch Southeast S8, B2, B8	Inner thighs and crotch (*gu* 股) Southeast, Wood, Wind, White "With regard to its application to people, it represents baldness, a broad forehead, and eyes with a lot of white area" 其於人也為寡髮為寡髮廣顙廣顙為多白眼.

best times to try to produce a baby, or perhaps it was meant to guide men in sexual cultivation practices.

One of the most colorful tales of a master healer is Tsinghua University bamboo manuscript *When Red Pigeons Gathered on Tang's House* (*Chijiu zhi ji Tang zhi wu* 赤鳩集湯之屋), featuring the minister Yi Yin, who specialized in soups and magic. Yi Yin, once possessed by a talking raven, gained super healing powers, thus reinforcing the Han tale of ancient doctors, like Bian Que, as being part bird (Unschuld, 2000, 64–65; Allan, 2015). As a chef, Yi Yin concocts a soup of the pigeons that had gathered on the roof of ruler Tang's house that allows the drinkers magical seeing powers (which the modern scholar Du Feng notes is similar to the "medicine for holding the center," *huizhong yao* 懷中藥, provided to the Lord of Changsang 長桑君 by Bian Que to cure the effects of old age: Du Feng, 2014a, 5; see *Shiji* 45). Yi Yin's cosmic knowledge (including the five flavors) is lauded in other Tsinghua bamboo manuscripts (Chen Hui 2019; Cook 2019; Guo Lihua 2019).

In *Red Pigeon*, the ruler Tang was angry that both Yi Yin and Tang's wife had tasted the soup before him. Yi Yin tried to run away, but Tang paralyzed him with a curse. A swarm of ravens spotted Yi Yin and thought about consuming him, but the chief, Shaman-raven (*wuwu* 巫烏), had another idea. He would possess Yi Yin's body and force him to travel to the competing political ruler, the emperor of the Xia, called Xia Hou 夏后 (who was doomed to be overthrown by Tang) and heal him of a heart problem. The cure was called "soothing the thorn-like pain" (*fu chu* 撫楚), possibly the name of a treatment or of a herb (Huang Dekun, 2013, 85 n. 17). Shaman-raven explained the demonic origins of the Lord of Xia's affliction:

> Di (the Sky god) commanded two yellow snakes and two white rabbits to take up residence in the beams of the lord's bedroom. They afflicted the lord underneath, causing a heart pressure disorder such that he did not recognize anyone. Di commanded the Earth god to make two mounds under the lord's bed that could jab the lord's body above, causing such evil turmoil that he could not rest

> 帝命二黃蛇與二白兔居后之寢之棟. 其下舍后疾是使后悗 (?)疾而不知人. 帝命后土為二陵屯, 其居后之牀下, 其上 斤 (析？刺?) 后之體是使后之身苟慝 不可及于席.

Yi Yin (possessed by the Shaman-raven) explained to Xia Hou that the house had to be demolished to expel the demonic manifestations (Allan, 2015, 5–8). The bodily symptom of "evil turmoil" (symptoms of demonic illness) occurs in other manuscripts (Huang Dekun, 2013, 86, n. 4; Li Ling in Ma Chengyuan, 2001–12, vol. 2, 276). Examples in the transmitted *Zuozhuan* and *Guoyu* point to the behavior of thieves, barbarians, and corrupt rulers. The paradigm for overthrowing a ruler is to end corruption and evil, as the king's body mirrored the health of the state.

Interestingly, this demonography is counterbalanced in the other Tsinghua bamboo texts featuring Tang, where we learn of his interest in the cosmic configurations of well-being. In the *Tang zai Chimen* 湯在啻門, for example, Yi Yin's explanation to Tang on the role of *qi* in life lays the ideological groundwork for Han sexual cultivation techniques and later medieval Daoist Inner Alchemy (*neidan* 內丹) practices that evolved under the influence of Buddhism into visualizing "embryos" of a pure self (Raz, 2014). Yi Yin explains that the embryo was the harmonious joining of the *qi* of the five flavors, initiated by the "jade seed, semen" (*yuzhong* 玉種). Ten months later, a baby was born. Although the heartbeat, amniotic sac, bones, muscles, and skin are mentioned, all other body terms are vague. This confirms the idea that it was only later that the five flavors begin to correspond to the five viscera. After the baby was born, it flourished as its *qi* expanded and become strong. Old age occurs as a result of slowing *qi* that goes in the wrong directions (*niluan* 逆亂), thus causing affliction. Death comes when *qi* reaches an end (*zhong* 終) and "the 100 intentions run out" (*baizhi er qiong* 百志而窮). The *Tang zai Chimen* contextualizes the creation of a human within the cosmic frame of state, Earth, and Heaven (see Cao Feng, 2019; Chen Hui, 2019; Cook, 2019; Guo Lihua 2019; Huang Guanyun, 2019).

The bamboo trigram divination text and the Tsinghua philosophical tales anticipate the view of the healthy human body as a microcosm of balanced cosmic influences but one that was still vulnerable to demonic forces. The correlative system of *yinyang wuxing* underpinning the transmitted canons is as yet unformed.

Qin Bamboo Texts: Magic and Recipes

As the Qin leaders swept east from their origins in the northwest beginning in the seventh century BCE, they forcibly mixed peoples and traditions from different cultural regions, culling from the knowledge network the technical expertise that they felt would be useful to run the empire they formed in the third century BCE. Divination and recipe texts were mixed with other types of technical information, such as sericulture, animal husbandry, astronomy, math, law, and much more. While medical information is diverse and mixed with magical formulas, we see a growing awareness of genres, such as women's and children's separate healing needs. We also see the emergence of named ailments, a distinction of the role of physician, and a tendency to consider clusters of symptoms – trends that continue during Han when medical literature begins to evolve as a separate genre.

Divination texts with medical predictions include (1) the hemerological "daybooks" (*rishu* 日書), found in sites in Shuihudi 睡虎地, Yunmeng 雲夢, Hubei (c. 217 BCE) and Fangmatan 放馬灘, Tianshui 天水, Gansu (ca. 239 BCE), and (2) other texts recovered from looters, such as the *Nine Stalks of Yu* (*Yu jiu ce* 禹九策), now preserved by Beijing University. Recipe texts include (1) fragments, also preserved in Beijing University, titled the *Random Jottings on Medical Recipes* (*Yifang zachao* 醫方雜抄) (ca. 214 BCE); (2) random strips lumped together with legal documents recovered from an ancient well at Liye 里耶, Changsha, Hunan (ca. 222–208 BCE), titled *Ailment Recipes* (*Bingfang* 病方); (3) Zhoujiatai (ca. 213–210 BCE) fragments titled *Recipes for Ailments and Other Things* (*Bingfang ji qita* 病方及其他). They are similar in style and content to Han recipe texts from MWD, LGS, and Han sites in Gansu: Wuwei and Dunhuang (Zhang Chaoyang, 2016, 68–69; Yang & Brown, 2017). Shared content from different regions and time periods helps scholars decipher and knit together fragmented strips as well as show how some treatments were transmitted over hundreds of years.

Daybooks reveal a continued concern with gender and time as factors for diagnosis and prognosis. They clarify the supernatural agency of the 10 Stems and 12 Branches signs, marking the days of the sexagenary calendar, the hours of the day, and their influence over the healing of the gendered body. The Qin further categorized the power of twelve differently named days linked to the movement of astral bodies such as the Dipper or the 28 Astral Lodges (*she* 舍) (Harper & Kalinowski, 2017, xxi–xxii, 139–142, 464–465). Such correlations with medical diagnoses appear in daybooks found in the tomb of a local official in Shuihudi. The section called "Sickness" (*bing*) is found in Daybook A between a section on a hemerological system called "stars" (*xing* 星) keyed to the twelve months and the 28 Astral Lodges and a list of good days for offering sacrifices to parents. In manuscript B, "Sickness" is only one line that appears between a section called "being afflicted" (*youji* 有疾) (with similar content to Sickness in A) and a section dealing with nightmares called "dreams" (*meng* 夢) (Harper & Kalinowski, 448, 452). Generally, illness is keyed to sexagenary days, directions, colors, and sometimes the Five Agents. What follows is a sample from manuscript A and Table 2 lists correlations in the section (Shuihudi Qin mu zhujian zhengli xiaozu, ed., 1990, 193). Note: "S#" = Stem, 1 through 10:

Sickness 病

    If you are afflicted on a Jia (S1) or Yi (S2) [day], then it is a curse from the parents that [must be resolved] with meat from the East wrapped up in a lacquer dish. Sickness will occur on a Wu (S5) or Ji (S6) [day] and recovery on a Geng (S7) [day], so express your gratitude through sacrifice on a Xin

Table 2 Daybook correlations

Days of affliction	Sources of curse	Days of sickness	Day of recovery	Day and items of sacrifice	Consequences and signs of death
S1 S2	Parents 父母	S5 S6	S7	S8, meat brought from the East wrapped up in a lacquer dish	Trouble (fever?), Year, East, Green
S3 S4	Grandfather 王父	S7 S8	S9	S10, red-colored meat, rooster, wine	Trouble, Year, South, Red
S5 S6	Shamans doing the *kan* (earth-pattern) walk (?) 巫措行 (or action by Shaman Kan), Grandmother 王母	S9 S10	S1	S2, yellow, *suo* 索 (dried?) fish, *qin* 堇 ale	Trouble in state center (*bang zhong* 邦中), Year in West (mistake for center?). Yellow
S7 S8	In-law ghosts (or others outside the clan) 外鬼, died of injuries 傷死	S1 S2	S3	S4, dog meat, fresh eggs, white	Trouble, Year, West, White
S9 S10	Strangers 毌逢人, in-law or non-kin ghosts 外鬼	S3 S4	S5	S6, ale, dried meat, strips of prepared meat	Trouble, Year, North, Black

(S8) [day]. If you don't then trouble will occupy the eastern (section of the residence) and the Year (astral spirit) will be in the East and [with the advent of] Green (in the cycle of Five Agents), death [will occur].

甲乙有疾父母為祟得之於肉從東方來裹以漆器. 戊己病庚有 (聞) 辛酢. 若不 [酢] 煩居東方歲在東方青色死.

The demonic sources of illness listed in Qin manuscripts are similar to those mentioned in the earlier *Stalk* and in a later early Han-period bamboo manuscript preserved by Beijing University self-titled as *Tricks of Jing* (*Jingjue* 荆決 (訣), hereafter *Tricks*). The difference is the names used for the numerical trigrams produced. The *Stalk* trigrams are gendered and link to names in the *Changes*, whereas the *Tricks* trigrams are named after select Stems and Branches (Cook & Zhao, 2017, 136–139; Dotson, Cook, & Zhao 2021, 163, 275–284). Gendered Stem and Branch signs appear in the Shuihudi daybooks and are used to mark a body diagram, but the correlation is different from the Chu system. In Qin and Han daybooks, the Branch signs only mark the periphery of the body and they rotate depending on the *yin* or *yang* nature of the season. Season, branch sign, and body section were correlated to calculate the fate of a pregnancy (Harper & Kalinowski, 2017, 244–247).

Daybooks also name some ailments that became categories of illness in Han medicine. One of thirty-three different ailments mentioned in the daybooks found in Fangmatan is *dan* 癉 ("exhaustion") (Yu Yue, 2015, 17–19). The tomb contents reflect a literate man concerned with fate. Besides daybooks, it also includes an account of a man resurrected from the dead, maps, and a Liubo 六博 game which could double as a cosmic divination board (Gansusheng wenwu kaogu yanjiusuo 2009). Strips 14 and 15 of Daybooks A and B record that on a "remove day" (*churi* 除日) (the second of the twelve day categories), people afflicted with *dan* would die.

Timing was critical to healing *dan* (see Zhoujiatai strip 313; Hubeisheng Jingzhoushi Zhouliang yuqiao yizhi bowuguan, 2001, 127; Chen Wei, 2005):

> In the first month select half a *sheng* measure of peach tree worm feces, add it to full-bodied ale, heat and drink it so people do not suffer an exhaustion (*dan*) ailment.
>
> 以正月取桃蠡 (蠹) 矢 (屎) 少半升, 置淳 (醇) 酒中, 溫, 飲之, 令人不單 (癉) 病.

In the *HDNJ* and MWD vessel texts, timing is not emphasized; *dan* is understood as heat experienced in a specific part of the inner body, such as the intestine (Zhang & Unschuld, 2015, 118; Harper 1998, 198). But in the LGS

Zhubing 諸病 2, it was caused by wind and, if afflicting the heart, linked to insanity (Wang Yitong, 2019, 18–21).

Fangmatan Daybooks A and B mention various odd physiognomic features, such as broken teeth, protruding eyes linked to big bellies, small necks or heads, black moles, and other physical "flaws, blemishes" (*ci* 疵). Daybook B mentions "suffering from illness" (*bing*) in a range of body parts (including heart, intestines, waist, kidneys, chest, ribs, shoulder, arms, neck, ears, eyes), often in combinations of body parts and connected with colors or physical attributes (strips 126, 90–107, 111, 113–121, 259). Han-period LGS texts reaffirm an attention to color. These correlations suggest an incipient interest in cosmological correspondences in which color reflects a quality of *qi* used in physiognomy (Despeux, 2005).

Removing or modulating physical defects is a shared concern in Qin and Han recipes (Harper 1998, 303). Zhoujiatai Strip 318 provides a technique for getting rid of black moles with a heat technique (Hubeisheng Jingzhoushi Zhouliang yuqiao yizhi bowuguan, 2001, 127–128; Wang Guiyuan, 2007):

> Recipe to get rid of black moles: select a small thin dried stalk, chop it up and gather [the pieces] together in a bundle about the size of the pinky finger. Select one *sheng* measure of gathered ashes and steep them [in ale], mix the stalk with the ashes, to rub on [the black moles] so the blood will come out. Then eat a lot of scallions so the sweat comes out. If they persist then select a lot of hoed-under mulberry wood [pieces] and burn them to ash; the slice up some beef about the size of the moles and cook it to ash [over the mole] so that it heats up but does not burn as it is applied to the black mole, when cold penetrates, do it over again.

> 去黑子方: 取稾本小弱者, 齊約大如小指. 取東 (棟) 灰一升, 漬之. 沭 (和) 稾本東 (棟) 灰中, 以靡 (摩) 之, 令血欲出. 因多食蔥, 令汗出. 柜 (恒) 多取 櫌桑木, 燔以為炭灰, 而取牛肉剤 (劙) 之, 小大如黑子, 而炙之炭火, 令溫 勿令焦, 即以傅黑子, 寒轍 (徹) 更之.

The divination manuscript titled the *Nine Stalks of Yu* seems to be a pastiche of fragments copied from earlier texts but with an added introduction and new commentary. The topic of illness is embedded in such concerns as travel, business, and proper sacrifice. The introduction explains that the two methods recorded involve the nine "stalks, counting rods" (*zhi* 支, read as *mei* 枚) of Yu and the five of Huangdi but does not display, as in the *Stalk* or *Tricks*, the mantic image (numerical trigram) of the results. In the *Changes* tradition, the number nine symbolized the peak of *yang* before it would flip to *yin*. In myth, nine also symbolized the Nine Continents of the earth. The number five was a *yang* number and could represent the *wuxing*. Huangdi symbolized celestial authority and Yu channeled the floods and healed the earth. In many Qin and Han recipe

Table 3 Numerical correlations and the body

Odd	Even
1: the right eye	2: left eye
3: right ear	4: left ear
5: right nostril	6: left nostril
7: anxious heart & grimacing mouth, two ears (of a vessel)	8: head & eyes (movement possibly related to turtle divination?)
9: the king's body	

texts, patients and healers had to perform am exorcism choreography called the Pace of Yu (*yubu* 禹步) to cure warts, hernias, abscesses, heart troubles, toothache, and more (Lewis, 2006b, 142–143). The body as a simulacrum of the earth's geography inspires Han vessel theory (Lo & Gu, in press).

In the Yu method, if odd numbers one, three, five, seven, or nine are thrown, the fortunes are generally auspicious; if even numbers two, four, six, or eight are thrown, they are inauspicious. The Huangdi sections, two each of good and bad fortunes, can be read as add-ons to the Yu sections, which are keyed by numbers and to parts of the body (mostly the face) but in a haphazard manner (Table 3).

The left side of the body is *yang* and the right *yin*. The text confirms a *yin*-and-*yang* correlation of number and time. If a six is thrown and you feel sick at midnight, this is inauspicious. Generally, illness in the Yu stalk sections is addressed only in terms of whether it is fatal or not. A few more specifics are found in the Huangdi sections. In the "Good Outcomes" (Shan 善) section, the text notes that affliction will be limited to the waist and spine (疾不在它方, 唯腰與脊) but that continuous sacrifices are necessary for the ailment of weakness (*wei bing*) to abate (今弗恆祠, 將瘣 (痿) 病弗舍). In the section "Bad Endings" (E *zhong* 惡終), skepticism creeps in:

> Praying and sacrificing unceasingly will have the same results as with a shaman or doctor. A person's fate will be such that prayers and sacrifices are of no use. Send away the shaman and release the doctor, retire to the bedroom, and prepare the articles for burial.
>
> 禱祠毋居, 巫醫是共. 命是將然, 祠祀奚攻 (功). 歸巫釋醫, 寢具葬庸.

The Huangdi passages above not only name a specific aliment, *wei*, but also make a purposeful distinction between two types of healers – shamans and doctors, specialists in invocations versus recipes, although clearly the arts overlapped. For the Qin, *wei* seems to be linked to supernatural affliction of the back, but in the transmitted texts it is understood as *bi* 痹 ("blocked *qi*") and linked to the inner body spaces (Tessenow & Unschuld, 2008, 2–24, 441–442). We see again a shifting focus from attention to the outer body to the inner body over time and represented in non-transmitted local manuscripts versus the edited canons.

There is a narrative similarity between the Huangdi "Good Outcomes" passage and the earliest documented use of *bi*, which occurs in a tale told by Xunzi in the third century BCE. Both passages reflect the popular conception that *bi* was the result of a person walking at night and running into a ghost. In the "Good Outcomes" passage, there is no question that it is a real ghost, but Xunzi claims the victim must have mistaken his own shadow for a ghost and just "lost his *qi* and died" (失氣而死). The transmitted Xunzi text (thus subject to later editing) goes on to explain the typical approach for healing this type of *bi*, which derives from dampness, not ghosts (translation adapted from Knoblock, 1988, vol. 3, 109):

> *Bi* is harm from dampness; in a case of *bi*, [people] beat drums and boil piglets, thus wasting money by wearing out drums and killing piglets, with no chance of curing the illness.

> 故傷於濕而痹, 痹而擊鼓烹豚, 則必有敝鼓喪豚之費矣, 而未有俞疾之福也.

Dealing with ghosts was a job for a "shaman" (*wu* 巫), a type of healer that can be traced back to OBI. The term "physician" (*yi* 醫) is relatively late. Qin daybooks suggest that a female might become either a shaman or a physician, but the latter role was considered bad luck for a female. It was good luck for a male to become a physician and "wear a cloak," a symbol of status (Shuihudi Qin mu zhujian zhengli xiaozhu, 1990, 252–253, Daybook B, strips 242, 244). In the Shuihudi legal texts, we find men and women of different status perform-ing "physical examinations" (*zhen* 診).

Two examples in the *Models for Sealing and Physical Examinations* (*Fengzhenshi* 封診式), a legal text found in the Shuihudi tomb, describe two diagnoses, one by a physician (presumably male) and the other by a bondswoman. The first concerns a specific ailment, a case of *li* 癘, which in this instance might be "leprosy" but elsewhere seems to be linked to seasonal pestilence, wind afflictions, insect infestations, or epidemics (translation adapted from McLeod & Yates, 1981, 152–153; Shuihudi Qin mu zhujian zhengli xiaozu, 1990, 156, strips 52–54):

> *Li* 癘
>
> Transcript: The Chief A of X village brought along villager C, a member of the rank and file. The denunciation reads: "I suspect [a case of] *li* and have come and brought him along. We questioned C. His statement reads: 'At the age of three, I became sick with sores on the head (病疕); my eyebrows

swelled up (眉突); it could not be ascertained what sickness it was. I have no other liability.' We ordered Physician D (醫丁) to examine him. D said: 'C has no eyebrows (無眉); the bridge of the nose is destroyed (艮本絕); his nasal cavity is collapsed (鼻空壞); if you prick his nose, he does not sneeze (嚏); elbows and knees down to the soles of both feet are defective and are suppurating in one place (肘膝 [] [] [] 到 [] 雨足下跨潰一所); his hands have no hair; I ordered him to shout and the *qi* of his voice was hoarse (令號其音氣敗). It is *li*.'"

Female servants familiar with women's issues and birthing are called in to diagnose a miscarriage for investigating officers (Barbieri & Yates, 2015, vol. 1, 150–152; translation adapted from McLeod & Yates, 1981, 159–160; Shuihudi Qin mu zhujian zhengli xiaozu, 1990, 161–162):

Aborted Child 出子
Transcript: The denunciation of A, the wife of a member of the rank and file of X village reads: "I, A, had been carrying a child for six months. Yesterday, [I, A] fought with adult female C, a fellow villager. A and C seized each other by the hair and C knocked A to the ground. The villager, *gongshi* D, came to the rescue and separated C and A. When A reached her house, she immediately became sick with belly pains (病腹痛); last night, the child miscarried and aborted (子變出)." Now A, having wrapped and carried the child, has brought it along to denounce herself and to denounce C. We immediately ordered the Foreman Clerk X to go and seize C and immediately to examine the sex of the baby, how much hair it had grown, and the appearance of the placenta (診嬰兒男女生髮及保之狀). We also ordered a bondswoman (*liqie* 隸妾) who has given birth several times (數字者) to examine the appearance of A's emissions of blood from her vagina and wounds (前血出及癰狀). We also questioned the people in A's house concerning the condition in which A reached the house and the type of belly pains when the child aborted.
Transcript of Assistant B: "[I] ordered the Foreman Clerk X and the bondservant X to examine the child which A had brought along. It had been previously wrapped in a cloth napkin and, in shape, it resembled clotted blood (衃血狀), large as a hand, and unidentifiable as a child. They immediately placed it in a basin of water and shook it: the clotted blood [became like] a child. Its head, body, arms, hands, fingers, legs down to the feet, and the toes, were of human type, but eyes, ears, nose, and sex were unidentifiable (其頭身臂手股以下到足足指類人而不可知目耳鼻男女). When it was taken out of the water, it again had the appearance of clotted blood."
Another Form for it reads: "We ordered the bondswomen X and Y, who have given birth several times, to examine A. They both stated that A had dried blood at the sides of her vagina (前旁有幹血). At the moment, blood is still being emitted, but it is lessening; it is not menses (朔事). X had been carrying a child but it miscarried (變). The blood on her vagina and the blood that is being emitted resembles A's."

While the physician interviews the patient and determines the ailment from a cluster of symptoms, the bondswoman draws on personal experience. Bondswomen were women forced into servitude as punishment for crimes committed by themselves or their male relatives such as assault (including fighting that caused a miscarriage) or theft (Barbieri & Yates, 196–198). It is possible, but unknown, that some served as midwives.

Shamans also helped with birthing. In an earlier mythological tale of the "birth" of Chu lineage identity (recorded in the fourth-century-BCE bamboo manuscript preserved at Tsinghua University and known as the *Chu ju* 楚居), the mother of the Chu ancestral founder died in childbirth (twins were born out her "side, ribs," *xie* 脅) while being attended to by a shaman (Cook & Luo, 2017). Despite these birthing tales, it would be centuries before the medical canons acknowledged the fields of gynecology and pediatrics (Furth, 1999; Wilms, 2005).

Physicians and legal secretaries used a variety of medical vocabulary in these passages: two types of sores, *bi* 疕 (head sore) and *yong* 癰 (wounds, abscess, used to describe a blood pattern in this case). Blood (*xue*) was discussed in terms of embryonic development (looking like blood clots, *pei* 坏), the "front" (genitals) (*qian* 前), and the menses (*shuo* 朔). Medical vocabulary is also recorded in the recipe texts, which were presumably recorded and consulted by physicians.

The recipe texts found among the 3,800 bamboo strips in layer 8 of Well no. 1 in Liye document a combination of pharmaceutical and magical approaches to healing. The following are two preserved on strip numbers 876, 1376, 1959, and on strip 1221 that show that physicians considered alternative methods for the same syndromes, such as sudden heart pain (*baoxin tong* 暴心痛) (Chen Wei, 2012, 293–294, 317–318; Zhang Chaoyang, 2016, 70–71; cf. Harper, 1998, 453; Brown, 2015, 80; Yang & Brown, 2017, 248):

> Recipe for curing sudden heart pain: Have (the patient) lean on the eaves of the left side of the house and with the left hand pluck stalks of foliage one *chi* (23.1 centimeters) long; do the Pace of Yu three times and break them and spread them on the patient's heart. According (to the type of patient), have the person (suffering in the) heart step with their left heel (dragging), (so for) males, 7 heel-down steps, for females, twice 7 heel-down steps. Already tested. No restrictions.

> 治暴心痛方：令以比屋左 [榮][以][左][手][操] 取其[木] [若] 草蔡長一尺, [禹][步]三析, 傅之病者心上。 因以做 (左?)足踐踵其心, 男子七踵, 女子 二七踵。 嘗試。 勿禁。

> (Recipe #) 7. Healing those suffering the burning sensation of sudden heart pain. Grind pennycress seeds. Grind two portions of 1 piece each of dried

ginger and a cinnamon twig. Grind them together. Once the three ingredients are blended together, extract a pinch the amount of three fingers up to the second joint and heat it in clarified ale.

七。病暴心痛灼灼者, 治之, 析蓂實, 冶, 二; 枯薑、菌桂, 冶, 各一。凡三物並和, 取三指撮到節二, 溫醇酒

Magical techniques found in both Qin and Han recipe texts include performing the Pace of Yu and some almost identical recipes (Harper, 1998, 167–169; Xie Minghong, 2018, 9–11; Wang Yitong, 2019, 32). In Zhoujiatai Strips 326–328 to cure toothaches, it is performed along with an invocation (Hubeisheng Jingzhoushi Zhouliang yuqiao yizhi bowuguan, 2001, 129; Harper & Kalinowski, 2017, 130–133):

Recipe for ending toothaches: look to the east at an old wall, perform the three steps of the Pace of Yu saying: "Ah! [I] dare report to the lord of the old wall to the east that X suffers from toothache and how to end X's toothache, [so I] offer [him] a black cow and calf." Look at a pottery tile and break it; look at a wall with tiles, then perform the Pace of Yu; when finished take a tile from the wall and bury it at the foot of the old wall to the east. Place the wall tile down [in the pit first, then] place the cows on top and cover it with the broken up tile, firmly burying them. Take the "cows" to be the "head bug" (i.e. the cause of the toothache).

已齲方: 見東陳垣, 禹步三步, 曰: "皋! 敢告東陳垣君子, 某病齲齒, 笱(苟) 令某齲已, 請獻驪牛子母." 前見地瓦, 操; 見垣有瓦, 乃禹步, 已, 即取垣瓦貍(埋) 東陳垣止(址) 下. 置垣瓦下, 置牛上, 乃以所操瓦蓋之, 堅貍(埋) 之. 所謂 "牛" 者, 頭虫也.

In another case (strips 335, 337, and 336; there is some debate regarding the order of these strips), the Pace of Yu, accompanied with an invocation to a mountain spirit, helps to heal a sick heart (Hubeisheng Jingzhoushi Zhouliang yuqiao yizhi bowuguan, 2001, 131; Wang Guiyuan, 2007):

Sufferers of heart ailments (should) perform the Pace of Yu three times and say: "Ha! (I) dare to report to Mt. Tai: To Mt. Tai so high, about a person who lives there, and to Elder [name missing], about a person who is resting on a mat, for no reason acquires a heart ailment, and for no reason gets worse." Then have the sufferers of heart ailments lie down with their head to the south and with their left foot tap two times seven. [take . . .] annually fruiting red locust with a single finger (or a single fingers worth of = a twig of?) and wave it over So-n-so's congested heart affliction, then with two hands wave it over the patient's abdomen.

病心者: 禹步三, 曰: 皋! 敢告泰山: 泰山高也, 人 [居之]。[] []之孟也, 人席之, 不智(知) 而心疾, 不智(知) 而咸戠。即令病心者南首臥, 而左足踐之二七。[something missing?] 歲實赤 [隁 (槐) 獨] 指, 擅某叚(瘕)心疾, 即兩手擅病者腹。

In this case, the affliction of the heart is described as *jia* 瘕 (congestion of *qi*). In later medical canons, this condition involves "painful abdominal nodes" or lumps that might move up or down with the *qi*, a type of "conglomeration illness" (Zhang & Unschuld, 2015, 244). We are reminded of Shao Tuo's affliction in the fourth century BCE.

Physicians may or may not have to consider time or gender restrictions. In Zhoujiatai strip 1397: "use one cup of warm wine to create the dosage; [depending on] the time period prohibit women eating pork" (以溫酒一桮和之到服藥 時禁女食彘肉). But, in some cases, time is not factored in, as on strip 1243: "If the cause of the illness is already known, heal it without regard to the season. Prepare enough of the healing herb to heal the illness. When already healed, wrap (the remaining) herb in cloth and store it. The method for curing is to expose it to sunlight until it is dry, (then) smith it" (病已如故, 治病毋時。壹治 藥足治病。藥已治, 裹以繒臧(藏)。治術暴(曝)若有所燥, 冶) (Chen Wei, 2012, 298–299).

Some Qin recipes were preserved in the Han. Liye and MWD recipes using similar dried and peeled herbs for "metal wounds" (Harper, 1998, 228; Fang & Hu, 2015). Zhoujiatai recipes (strips 309–310) for "intestinal flushing" (*changpi* 腸澼), possibly dysentery, are also comparable (Hubeisheng Jingzhoushi Zhouliang yuqiao yizhi bowuguan, 2001, 126–137; Zhang & Unschuld, 2015, 80; Harper, 2010, 56–58; Fang & Hou, 2015, 52–53):

> Select the gall-bladder of a fat bovine and stuff it with black beans and the string it up and hang it in a dark place to dry out. To use it, remove 10 or so beans, put them in congee and drink it to end intestinal flushing (*changpi*). If it doesn't end, drink more of it again. With ingesting enough congee, the intestines . . . .

> 取肥牛膽盛黑叔 (菽) 中, 盛之而係 (系), 縣 (懸) 陰所, 幹. 用之, 取十餘叔 (菽) 置鬻(粥) 中而飲之, 巳 (已) 腸辟 (澼). 不已, 復益飲之. 鬻 (粥) 足以入 之腸 . . . .

Treating heat ailments is common in both time periods. For example, on Zhoujiatai Strip 311 we find: "For those who suffer a warmth ailment but don't sweat, soak a cloth in full-bodied ale, drink it" (溫病不汗者, 以淳 (醇) 酒漬布, 飲之) (Hubeisheng Jingzhoushi Zhouliang yuqiao yizhi bowuguan, 2001, 126; Fang & Hou, 2015, 53–54; Xie Minghong, 2018, 31–32; in MWD, Harper, 1998, 453). The influence of seasonal or geographical hot and cold agencies begins to emerge during the Han. More than a millennium later, exposure to heat in southern climates was considered a source of epidemics (Hanson, 2011).

The Beijing University manuscript *Random Jottings on Medical Recipes* was written on the back of a bamboo roll (*juan*), behind a mathematical calculation text for land measurement (the *Suan shu* 算書) and on the same roll as the *Nine Stalks of Yu* discussed earlier. Like Shuihudi manuscripts (and even many paper codices in the medieval Dunhuang collection), a bricolage of vaguely technical texts had been copied onto both sides of the manuscript. These included daybooks and texts on roads, clothing, and exorcism (Tian Tian, 2017, 52–53). The medical fragments reveal no obvious order and mix human conditions with silkworm problems (Tian Tian, 2017, 55–57). In the samples that follow, afflictions such as heart pain, seizures, and intestinal flushing are treated with magical techniques such as spitting and invocation, as well as with recipes, many using ingredients such as menstrual cloths. Han recipes treat the same afflictions with similar styles of treatments but with varied ingredients (Harper, 1998, 163–166, 246–247, 261, 282; Beijing daxue chutu wenxian yanjiusuo, 2013, 37–39).

> For heart affliction, invoke, spit, and say: "Tok! Father and mother of So-n-so do not account for time in the case of So-n-so causing him endless heart pain; make him spit at it."

> 祝心疾唾之曰: 歇, 某父某母為某不以時, 令某心痛毋期, 令某唾之.

> For a case of one afflicted with madness (or seizures?) where internal leaking blood will not come out, rinse out a young woman's menstrual cloth in a cup of water and drink it.

> 瘨 (癲?) 而內漏血不出者, 以女子月事布, 水一桮 (杯), 濯之而飲.

> For a case of intestinal flushing, select a good section of rice stalk and grind it up finely, boil up some of it in rice water and drink it without eating anything.

> 腸辟 (澼), 取稻米善簡析摩, 取其泔埶 (熟) 煮之而飲之, 毋食它物.

Herbs and magical treatments are applied to abscesses, itchiness, heart pain, blocked urine, as well as issues having to do with childbirth and childcare. In an example of how to heal an abscess (strip 16), "pick the root of *lian* 薟 (*Ampelopsis japonica*), wash off the dirt and grind it up with salt, mix in a little rice rinse water and apply it [to the affected area]. Remove it after one night" (已癰, 取薟本, 洗去其土, 以鹽庿之, 以沐少和之, 即以涂之, 壹宿而去之). On strip 32, there appears another recipe for treating "abscesses that are festering, use pig, sheep, and chicken excrement [mixed] with Yanlu (an herb) and pig's fat, and heat it [over the afflicted area] until the end of the day, and stop" (癰潰者, 以豕矢, 羊矢, 雞矢, 奄盧, 豕膏, 熏之冬 (終) 日, 已矣). For a fussy baby (strips 2 and 11): "if you carry an infant with you when you are guest in someone's home and the infant won't stop hollering, have someone take the infant's left hand and shake it ... enter the room, do it (like grinding something in a mortar?) in two [sets of] seven times and there will be no more hollering" (負嬰兒爲人客, 嬰兒篤虒 (嗁) 不可止. 令人把嬰兒左手, 以搖, … 入室, 曰二七, 不虒 (嗁) 矣). Similar recipes can be found in Zhoujiatai, Liye, and MWD (Tian Tian, 2017, 53–54). The numerical sets of seven are also found in the ZJS manuscripts.

As we saw with Xia Hou's bedroom in the analysis of *When Red Pigeons Gathered on Tang's House* and also occurring in the Baoshan record discussed earlier, living spaces could be demonically infested and cause illness. The Qin exorcism includes a special herb, Pig's Head (also known as Tianmingqing 天名精, *Carpesium abrotanoides*), as well as invocation. For example, see strips 18–20 (Tian Tian, 2017, 54–55):

> On the first Mao Day (B4) in the first month, pick 3 [stalks of?] Pig's Head, gather it in a bouquet and grind it up, purify it with ale, and toss the sediment into the well, using the juice to sacrifice at the doors of the gate and the four corners of the residence. Invoke (spirits with a spell): "God (*di*) has a divine herb named Pig's Head, born in winter, flourishing in summer, sharing God's chamber; drink it to expel the 100 afflictions; elder father and elder mother, do not let the 100 afflictions pass through So-n-so's chamber." Drink it without eating and at first step forward [three times (?)].

> 正月上卯, 取豕首三、韋束一, 薺(齏)之, 以酉(酒)淳之, 而投其宰(滓)井中, 以其汁祭門戶、宮四陋. .祝曰:"啻(帝)有神草, 名爲豕首, 冬生夏實, 與啻(帝)同室, 飲之以去百疾, 丈父丈母, 毋令百疾過某室。"飲之, 毋庸食, 先少(步)者(?)始(?)。

The call for father and mother spirits to intervene is found in the MWD *Recipes* as part of incantations to relieve "urine retention" (*long*) and "inguinal swelling" (*tui* 癩) (Ma Jixing, 1992, 477; Harper, 1998, 162, 259–263).

The Qin also continued the late Zhou practice of praying to nature spirits to heal illness. An inscription on both sides of two jade plaques of unknown provenance but presently stored in the Shanghai Museum has been the source of much scholarly speculation, particularly since many words are hard to decipher (Hou Naifeng, 2005). The inscription (side 1 is carved into the jade; sides 2–4 are written in red ink) can be generally understood to be as follows:

> Side 1: A descendant and heir of the Qin [royal family] Yin said: It is mid-winter, month 11, and the retreating *qi* (results in) harmful withering. My body has encountered an illness which makes me depressed. Tossing and turning with anxiety, there is no improvement, no cure. Nobody understands it and neither do I and so it remains completely uncertain. I am at my wits end as to what to do and full of fear and despair.

又(有)秦曾孫小子騆曰: 孟冬十月, 厥氣 [] (敗? 戕?) 週 (凋). 余身曹 (遭) 病, 為我憾憂. [] [] 反 [] (側), 無間無瘳. 眾人弗智 (知), 余亦弗智 (知), 而 靡有鼎 (定?息?) 休. 吾窮而無奈之可 (何), 永戁憂螯 (愁).

Side 2: The Zhou era is gone, with its statues and laws scattered and lost. Oh dear, I, the Little One, wish to serve Heaven and Earth, the Four Pivots, the Three Brilliances, the Mountains and Rivers, the spirits (above and below), the Five Annual Sacrifices, the Founding Ancestors, but have no access to their methods. Presenting fine sacrificial male-pigs and exquisite jades and silks, I, the descendant, feel so confused and blundering.

周世既沒, 典瀍 (法) 蘚 (散) 亡, 惴惴小子, 欲事天地, 四亟 (極), 三光, 山 川, 神示 (祇), 五祀, 先祖, 而不得厥方. 羲 (犧) 豝既美, 玉帛 (?) 既精, 余毓 子厥惑, 西東若惷.

Side 3: There is a man from the east who handles punishments and law (or methods for natural configurations?), his name is Xing. He is pure when it comes to methods and clean when it comes to doing the right thing. I dare to announce: "I am innocent! [please] make the spirits understand my situation"; it's as if the spirits do not accept one's actions and [insist on] punishing the innocent (?), who among the loyal (?) people serving the spirits [then] dare not be true?

東方有士姓, 為刑 (形?) 瀍 (法) 氏, 其名曰陘. 潔可以為瀍 (法), 淨 (?) 可 以為正. 吾敢告之: 余無辜 (罪) 也, 使明神智 (知) 吾情; 若明神不 [] 其行, 而無辜 (罪) [] 友 (宥?) 刑 (?), [] [] [] (烝) 民之事明神, 孰敢不精?

Side 4: I, Little One Yin, dare to take up a large jade scepter, an auspicious jade circlet, and auspicious jade [horse ornament?] to report to the Great Mountain Hua: "Great Mountain, grant me in the eighth month to return the illness afflicting my body (heart and abdomen) and legs (lower and upper sections of the legs) to its origin. Please take charge of the jades and use the two just seven-year-old bovine sacrificial animals, the purified X and goats, pigs, four chariot horses, three people from a single household who come forward with one jade circlet to walk along the dark and light sides of Great Mountain Hua to mitigate the spiritual blame. Once the spiritual blame is mitigated ... then they will bury (the sacrificial objects) to the glory of their descendants for myriad generations. If [you, Great Mountain] cause my, the Little One Yin's, illness to revert to its origin, [I shall] report it to Taiyi and the Great General, and so too will the family (of the people sacrificed?) and the royal household (report it).

小子騆敢以芥 (介, 玠) 圭, 吉璧, 吉 [] 以告於 [] (華) 大山. 大山又(有) 賜, 八月(?) 已吾 (?) [] (腹) 心以下至於足髀之病能自復如故. 請又 (有?) 司 [], (?) 用牛羲 (犧) 貳, 亓(其) 齒七, 潔 (?) [] [] 及羊, 豢, 路車四馬, 三人壹家, 壹璧先之; [] [] 用貳羲 (犧), 羊, 豢, 壹璧先之, 而 [] (覆) [] (華) 大山之陰陽, 以遂 (?) 悠 (?) 㝊, 悠 (?) 㝊既 [], 其XX裡, 枼 (世) 萬子孫, 以此為尚 (常). 句 (茍) 令小子騆之病日 (自?) 復故, 告太一, 大將軍, 人壹家 (?), 王室相如.

The patient, Yin, believed to be King Hui Wen of Qin 秦惠文王 (r. 325–311), felt anxiety and pain in his upper and lower body and accused a spirit, possibly Hua Mountain (or a nature spirit under its authority), of afflicting him in retaliation ("spiritual blame," *jiu* 咎) for ending the Zhou era. Hua Mountain (the sacred peak of the west versus Taishan, the sacred peak of the east) seems to be under the authority of star spirits, Taiyi and the Great General. To intercede with this powerful pantheon, Yin used an occult specialist from the East (Chu? Yue?) to direct the sacrificial ritual and get the spirits to take back their curse. The notion of spiritual blame causing illness goes back to the Shang; the term *jiu* is common in late Zhou texts (Cook, 2006, 80–81). In Chu records, mountain deities were among the many spirits considered as possible culprits (or as possible sources of salvation), who must be offered animal and other sacrifices.

Qin medical manuscripts bridge the transition from the performance of purely magical medicine to a focus on collecting recipes for healing specific conditions. Magical medicine reflects the continued belief in perverse external influences – supernatural and increasingly environmental – over human health. Attention to the inner versus just the external body condition is reflected in the increase in diagnosing clusters of symptoms as named ailments. There is also evidence of increased professionalism and the use of a variety of approaches to treat both ailments and symptoms. A fuller imagination of the inner body landscape emerges during the Han.

Han Bamboo and Silk Manuscripts: Medical Literature As a Genre

The bamboo and silk manuscripts discovered in Mawangdui, Changsha, Hunan (MWD), in the early 1970s revolutionized our understanding of ancient medicine. The tomb includes a range of medical literature along with manuscripts on philosophy and "technical arts" (*shushu* 數術), maps, and charts (Ma Jixing, 1992; Harper, 1998). Healing the sick body and enhancing the healthy were cojoined arts. A similar mix of recipe, magical, vessel-theory, and nurturing long-life (*yangsheng*) texts was found in a tomb in Zhangjiashan, Hubei (ZJS). This tomb also included legal, mathematical, divination, and other technical arts texts, but no philosophical texts. Scattered Han medical writings have also been found in the medieval Buddhist caves at Dunhuang in Gansu and in a watchtower in Juyan 居延, Ejina 額濟納, Mongolia (99 BCE–31 CE). Recipe and other bamboo texts (comprising about 900 strips) were discovered in second-century-BCE Han burials in 2012–13 in Chengdu, Sichuan (Laoguanshan), along with a remarkable inscribed lacquerware figure. Later Han (mid-first-century-CE) materials include bamboo texts discovered in the early 1970s from a tomb in Wuwei, Gansu (Yang & Brown, 2017).

In the family graveyard of the local ruler of Changsha Kingdom, Li Cang 利蒼 (d. 186 BCE), in tomb no. 3, the tomb of Li's thirty-year-old son (d. 168 BCE) contained a lacquer box filled with about thirty manuscripts along with maps, diagrams, and pictures (Harper, 1998, 14–16). Of these, sixteen are classed as medical literature (Mawangdu Han mu boshu zhenli xiaozu, 1985). Three of them had two versions (Ma Jixing, 1992, 4–5). From their script styles and vocabulary, scholars assume they represent copies of texts actually written at different times, some as early as the Qin (Ma Jixing, 1992, 8–21; Harper, 1998, 19–30, 38–40). Some are versions of texts also found in ZJS, suggesting a shared knowledge circulated by specialists. One of the most significant advances that these texts represent is the documentation of vessel theory (but only numbering eleven vessels and not the twelve recorded in the *HDNJ*). There is no evidence of acumoxa. The texts note the lancing of swellings on the body but only cauterization to treat the vessels (Harper, 1998, 5). This contrasts with later canonical literature.

The MWD library of medical literature is fundamental to our understanding of Han practice. The texts, listed below, were all titled by modern archaeologists; the title translations and notes about which texts are grouped together are drawn from Donald Harper (1998):

(1) The following texts share one large silk 24 × 450 centimeters long (sections of these texts, except for the last, *Recipes*, are also found in the ZJS *Maishu*; see Lo, 2000, 18–19):

> *Cauterization Canon of the Eleven Vessels of the Foot and Forearm* (*Zubi shiyi mai jiujjing* 足臂十一脈究經)
> *Cauterization Canon of the Eleven Yin and Yang Vessels* (*Yinyang shiyi mai jiujing* 陰陽十一脈灸經) (Versions A & B)
> *Model of the Vessels* (*Maifa* 脈法) (Versions A & B)
> *Death Signs of the Yin and Yang Vessels* (*Yinyang mai sihou* 陰陽脈死候) (Versions A & B)
> *Recipes for Fifty-two Ailments* (*Wushier bingfang* 五十二病方)

(2) The following texts share one large silk approximately 50 × 110 centimeters long:

> *Eliminating Grain and Eating Vapor* (*Quegu shiqi* 却穀食氣)
> *Cauterization Canon of the Eleven Yin and Yang Vessels* (*Yinyang shiyi mai jiujing* 陰陽十一脈灸經)
> *Drawings of Guiding and Pulling* (*Daoyin tu* 導引圖)

(3) On a single badly damaged silk approximately 24 centimeters wide:

> *Recipes for Nurturing Life* (*Yangsheng fang* 養生方)

(4) On another badly damage silk of about the same size:

Recipes for Various Cures (*Zaliao fang* 雜療方)

(5) On a silk 49 × 49 centimeters:

Book of the Generation of the Fetus (*Taichan shu* 胎產書)

(6) On 33 bamboo slips:

Ten Questions (*Shiwen* 十問)
Conjoining Yin and Yang (*He yinyang* 合陰陽)

(7) On 11 wooden slips:

Recipes for Various Charms (*Zajin fang* 雜禁方)

(8) On 56 bamboo slips:

Discussion of the Culminant Way in Under-heaven (*Tianxia zhidao tan* 天下至道談)

Ma Jixing (1992, 3–4) divides the texts into four main types: preventative medicine (including some self-cultivation texts), medical theory (vessel and cauterization as well as some self-cultivation texts), therapeutic (recipe and some of the vessel and cauterization texts), and other (including self-cultivation sex texts, charms, spells, and magical techniques). He notes a number of categories of ailments, including: "injury" (*shang* 傷), "spasms" (*xian* 癇), "urine retention" (*long*), "hemorrhoids" (*zhi* 痔), "abscesses" (*yong*), "festering pustules" (*ju* 疽), "scabbing" (*bi*), "scabies" (*jia* 痂), "facial pustules" (*ma* 瘙), and others of unsure meaning (Ma Jixing, 1992, 28; translations adapted from Harper, 1998; Zhang & Unschuld, 2008).

The locations of the eleven vessels and sets of syndromes are described in the cauterization manuals but not always in a uniform manner. Basically, there are sets of *yin* and *yang* vessels that originate in the feet and hands and thread their way around muscles and bone into the core of the body or up to the head. They were not interconnected as described in the *HDNJ* (Harper, 1998, 82–90; he suspects that the use of *yin* and *yang* initially referred to relative inner or outer sides of muscles around which the vessels moved). The two sets of vessels include Great Yang (*taiyang* 太陽), Minor Yang (*shaoyang* 少陽), Yang Brilliance (*yangming* 陽明), Minor Yin (*shaoyin* 少陰), Great Yin (*taiyin* 太陰), and Ceasing Yin (*jueyin* 厥陰) vessels, although the *jueyin* vessel for the hands is missing from the MWD corpus. Viscera, such as heart, stomach, liver, and spleen, are mentioned but without the systematic correlations described in the *HDNJ*. The term *wuzang liufu* (five viscera and six cavities) appears only in a self-cultivation context involving the technique

Table 4 Body formation correlations

Month	Agent	Body
4	Water	Blood
5	Fire	*Qi*
6	Metal	Muscle
7	Wood	Bone
8	Earth	Skin
9	Stone	Hair

of "sucking *qi*" (*xiqi* 噏氣) in the *Ten Questions*. In the *HDNJ*, the hand Great Yin vessel reaches the lungs. In the MWD texts, it reaches the heart. On the other hand, the kidney is mentioned in connection to the foot Minor Yin vessel in the *Cauterization Canon of the Eleven Yin and Yang Vessels* (hereafter *Yinyang*) as well as in the *HDNJ* (Harper, 1998, 210).

In the MWD text *Book of the Generation of the Fetus*, the *wuxing* are correlated with time as seen in Qin daybooks (not viscera as in *HDNJ*). Interestingly, whereas in the late Zhou *Stalks* manual there were only four agents, in the MWD text there are six, each correlated with a month numbering four to nine and a developing part of the fetus (Harper, 1998, 379–380) (Table 4). The *Changes* tradition of odd-*yang*, even-*yin* numbers seems to inform these correlations. In the MWD vessel texts, *yin* vessels indicate death and the *qi* of Earth versus *yang* vessels with life and the *qi* of Heaven (Harper, 1998, 88).

Ma Jixing (1992, 89) notes the great variability in the vessel paths described in MWD versus *HDNJ*. The MWD hand *yin* vessels go from the hands to the chest, but in *HDNJ* the direction of influence is the opposite. The MWD hand *yang* vessels go from hands to head just like the *HDNJ*, except for the MWD Great Yang vessel, which goes from head to hand. The MWD foot *yin* vessels go from foot to thighs to abdomen in one text (*Cauterization Canon of the Eleven Vessels of the Foot and Forearm*, hereafter *Zubi*) and from head to abdomen in another (*Yinyang*), except for the Great Yin vessel, which went from lower abdomen to the foot. The foot *yin* vessels in the *HDNJ* go from foot to chest. The foot *yang* vessels go from the malleolus or shin to the head in one text (*Zubi*) or to the thigh or head in another (*Yinyang*). In the *HDNJ*, they go from head to feet.

Ma Jixing (1992, 26) notes a few areas used for pulse-reading: above the inner malleolus, along the Minor Yin vessel of the lower body, and along the Great and Minor Yang vessels of the arms. The qualities of pulse determined

were listed in the *Model of the Vessels* (*Maifa*) and in the ZJS *Maishu*: "full"
(*ying* 盈), "empty" (*xu* 虚), "slippery" (*hua* 滑), "rough" (*se* 濇 or 澀), and
"quiet" (*jing* 靜) (Ma Jixing, 1992, 295; Hsu, 2010, 31). The *Maifa* explains:

> The way to examine the vessels: Place the left [hand five *cun* (about 11 cm) up
> from the malleolus] and press on it (*an* 案). Place the right hand at the malleolus
> and palpate it (*tan* 撣). If other vessels are full and this one alone is empty, it
> controls the ailment. If other vessels flow evenly (slippery) and this one alone is
> blocked (rough), it controls the ailment. If other vessels are still and this one
> alone is agitated, it controls the ailment. (after Harper, 1998, 216–217)

The physician diagnoses by pressing or palpating different vessels to evaluate
their relative fullness and texture of flow.

Pathology arises when a vessel is "moved, disturbed" (dong 動) or experi-
ences a "reversal" (*jue* 厥) (Harper, 1998, 202). For example, if the foot Yang
Brilliance vessel is moved, a person may shiver with cold, yawn and stretch
a lot, have swellings, have extreme anxiety, or maybe even run around singing
without clothing. Pain and numbness in different parts of the body linked
together by a vessel explain seemingly diverse symptoms (Ma Jixing, 1992,
232–238; Harper, 1998, 206). In heat illnesses, for example, we see that
treatments vary according to the vessel affected and whether it was a *yin* or
yang one, or a mixture of *yin* and *yang* vessels – suggesting that reading the
combined *yin*-and-*yang* signature of the body is not conceptually unlike reading
the lines of a *Changes* hexagram. If a patient has five or more of the symptoms
linked to the Ceasing Yin vessel of the foot, they will die, unless a *yang* vessel is
also involved. Ailments arising in connection with more than one vessel factor
into the outcome.

Heat illnesses mentioned include those that are internal (*zhong*), cause sweat-
ing, or a "troubled heart (delusions accompanying fever?)" (*fanxin* 煩心) – a
symptom often indicating psychological symptoms and severity. Related afflictions are coldness syndromes, some which cause shaking or alternate with hot
(*nüe*) (Ma Jixing, 1992, 29). The texts instruct the physician to cauterize the Great
Yang or Yang Brilliance vessels of the foot for coldness experienced in the middle
of the forehead but the Minor Yang of the foot for a cold shin. For heart trouble,
cauterize the foot Ceasing Yin vessel. If heart trouble is combined with belching
(evidence of rising *qi*), then cauterize the forearm Great Yin vessel.

In the *HDNJ*, vessels are treated with needling or moxibustion through
"openings" (*xue* 穴, *qiao* 竅, *kou* or *cunkou* 寸口) but these terms do not appear
in the MWD corpus. When the term "Nine Apertures" (*jiuqiao*) does appear, it
refers not to points on the body but to actual openings in the body – mouth, ears,
eyes, nostrils, genitals, or anus – that *qi* could penetrate to fill the inner body

(*zhong*) or the Six Cavities (*liufu*). It is not clear where on the body the physicians who used the MWD literature treated the vessels. In some cases, it seems to be around the waist, possibly to redirect the movement of *qi* (Harper, 1998, 91). There is evidence for the strategic use of lancing stones (*bian* 砭) and heat through cauterization (*jiu* 灸). Heat therapies included roasting the afflicted area over fire, pressing hot objects against it, fumigating it, or soaking it in a hot medicinal bath (Harper, 1998, 95–97). Other therapies included "pulling" (*yin*, guiding the *qi* through physical contortions) and massage, superficial surgery, drugs, and magic (Harper, 1998, 395; Lo, 2018b, 76).

The overlapping goals of healing and self-cultivation are evident from manuscripts and texts found in MWD and elsewhere (Li Jianmin, 2007, 146–190). The "Pulling" manuscripts discovered at MWD (including the *Daoyintu* and others) and ZJS (*Yinshu*) describe an exercise culture in which physical postures, named after wild animals, helped strengthen areas of the body and in some cases healed by pulling or guiding out the sources of pain, such as internal heat (Harper, 1998, 312–315; Lo, 2018b, 84–86). The physical choreography required is reminiscent of exorcistic movements used in healing. For example, to heal exhaustion (*dan*), the ZJS manual, strip 29, advises (after Lo, 2014, 38–40):

> Pulling inner exhaustion: Squat and [do something] with the buttocks, with the left hand stroke the neck, with the right hand stroke the left hand, raise the yoke of the neck (?) and bend forward as far as possible, then slowly in a relaxed manner focus on exhaling (the source of the exhaustion). Straighten up, raise the head and stop. (Once) settled down, then repeat five times.

> 引內癉：危坐 [] 尻，左手撫頸，右手撫左手，上扼(?)俯極，因徐縱而精呴之，端仰而已，定右復之五而。。。

Healing and strengthening the body also included sexual practices. In *Conjoining Yin and Yang*, a female orgasm helps the male to absorb *yin qi* to balance excess inner *yang qi* (Lo, 2000, 23; Lo, 2013, 2018a). Vivienne Lo's investigations of two lacquerware figurines discovered in Han coffins in Sichuan suggest that vessel therapy combined healing with longevity goals such as achieving a "jade body" (Lo & He, 1996; Lo, 2000; Lo & Gu, in press). They do not appear to be gendered, attesting to Charlotte Furth's theory of the generally androgynous approach to medicine before the Chao Yuanfang's and Sun Simiao's introduction of gynecology in the medieval era (Furth, 1999). These small probably handheld sculptures, one from Shuangbaoshan 雙寶山 and one from LGS, like the MWD texts, depict eleven vessels that run in parallel lines from the feet and hands up through the body into the head.

The vessel pattern on the figure from LGS is the more complex of the two. The following observations are drawn from brief reports, photographs, and personal observation of the artifact in the Chengdu museum. Vessels are depicted in two different colors, white and red, and some intersect, looping across others over the shoulder blades and creating a loose network across the front torso and abdomen area, roughly dividing it into three regions corresponding to the upper, middle, and lower burners (*jiao* 焦). Inscribed terms may coincide with acumoxa points. Notably five viscera are inscribed in a line down the spine, beginning at the top: heart, lungs, liver, stomach, and spleen. (The *HDNJ* includes the kidneys, not the stomach, in the *wuzang*.) The backs of the figure's knees are called *xi* 奚 (溪 "streams") (Lo & Gu, in press). At the front of the body, over the clavicle, is the "basin" (*pen* 盆), a well-known term. Down over the right breast, next to a hand vessel, is an unknown graph. It is positioned like the modern Pericardium meridian or the Ceasing Yin hand vessel missing in MWD. The graph resembles *yun* 氳 (a primal earth *qi*)*, hu* 壺 (vase-type ale vessel), *yi* 壹 (one), or *yun* 壹 (another way of writing primal earth *qi*) (Ke & Cai, 2021). The point near it on the Pericardium meridian would be PC-1 Celestial Pool (Tianchi 天池), which in the *HDNJ* is described as along the "hand-heart ruler [conduit]" (Unschuld, 2016a, 70). The term *yun* does not appear in the *HDNJ*. In the MWD and ZJS vessel texts, the earth *qi* links to *yin*, perhaps suggesting the vessel type (Harper, 1998, 79; Lo, 2000, 26–28). Clearly visible down the right side of the trunk is the term "armpit abyss" (*yeyuan* 腋淵). In fact, the term appears in reverse, *yuanye*, in the *HDNJ* as a point near the "big network [vessel] of the spleen" before it spreads to the chest and flanks (Unschuld, 2016a, 208; now it is along the Gall Bladder meridian, GB-22). There may be still other inscriptions on the body to be discovered once official photographs are formally published.

The practice of needling is evident in second-century-BCE Sichuan and also later in Gansu. The first-century-CE medical manuscripts discovered in a vaulted tomb in Wuwei, Gansu, include recipes, *materia medica*, and acupuncture therapy. The time-contingent acupuncture treatment prohibitions link early concerns with later medieval practices (Yang & Brown, 2017, 241, 245, 249). Recipes for decoctions follow ailment descriptions, a tradition also tracing back to the Qin. The recipes are general cures or for specific ailments such as persistent coughs (*jiu kai shang qi* 久欬上氣), cold damage following wind exposure (*shanghan sui feng*), metal wounds, eye pain, large accumulations in the heart and abdomen (*xinfu daji* 心服大積), chronic diarrhea (*jiu xie* 久泄), male sexual deficiencies, abscesses, scabs, and *qi* reversal (*niqi* 逆氣) syndromes including throat paralysis, heart and abdominal pain, throat pain, uterine pain, dry throat, and tooth pain (Yang & Brown, 2017, 258–301).

Of particular interest is the section on strips 19–23 that detail needling rules for particular ailments – for example, where to position the needle, how deep, and how long to keep it there. It also cites prohibitions by age and location of the body from a lost text *Huangdi's Prohibitions Regarding the Souls When Curing Illness* (*Huangdi zhibing shenhun ji* 皇帝治病神魂忌). The prohibitions restrict the needling or cauterizing of areas of the body that are occupied by souls at certain ages. This idea of souls moving around the body according to the calendar or age is prevalent in medieval texts discovered at Dunhuang (Harper, 2005; Despeux, 2007). In the Wuwei manuscript, the key locations are the heart (age one), the abdomen (age two), the back (age three), the head (age four), the feet (age five), hands (age six), shins (age seven), shoulders (age eight), [missing text]. People aged between 60 and 70 are treated the same as 6-year-olds; those between 70 and 80 as 7-year-olds; those between 80 and 90 as 8-year-olds; and those between 90 and 100 as 9-year-olds. People over 100 should not be needled or cauterized at all because the *qi* vessels are completely "cut off" (*qi mai yi jue* 氣脈壹絕) (Yang & Brown, 2017, 267–268). Prohibitions by Stem and Branch day listed on wooden tablets also determine treatments and link the late Han practice back in time to Qin daybooks. In the Wuwei text, on a Chen (B5) or Xin (S8) day, one cannot cauterize, needle, or drink decoctions. New moons and dark nights as well as Jia (S1) and Wu (B7) are also dangerous (Yang & Brown, 2017, 299–300).

In general, we see Han medicine as a continuation of Qin concerns but with new trends developing. There is an increasing interest in development and archiving of medical literature. There is a growing tendency to incorporate aspects of cosmic medicine with the magical, although a concern with the supernatural influence of time is common to both practices. Acumoxa practices and rudimentary *yinyang wuxing* correlations become evident in texts found in the west. Healing and self-cultivation were joined arts to maintain physical and mental welfare. In general, we see the seeds of approaches laid out in the canons but little evidence of a predominant canonical literature guiding physicians.

Medieval Paper Texts: The Persistence of Magic

The legacy and transformation of Han medicine through Silk Roads contacts are evident in the thousands of texts discovered in the early twentieth century that had been stashed in Buddhist Cave 17 at Dunhuang sometime in the eleventh century. Seventy-four medical texts were found; as in Qin and Han texts, medieval medical texts shared a single book or codex with a wide range of other types of text (Wang & Barrett, 2005). Many are Tang copies of earlier texts or even ancient originals. Ma Jixing (1988) categorizes the medical texts as:

(1) versions of chapters found in the *HDNJ* on the signs of death and pulse-taking;

(2) three variations of viscera or *wuzang* theory, presumably based on the theories of Mingtang (Illuminated Hall), Zhang Zhongjing (Han physician), and Jīvaka (Qipo 耆婆) (fifth-century-BCE doctor of Buddha);

(3) diagnostic methodologies that are mostly types of pulse-reading, but other methodologies such as divination as well;

(4) cold damage theory, some similar to material found in the transmitted *Shanghan lun* and the *Jingui yaolüe fanglun*;

(5) treatments, including secret instructions (from a ghost) on the internal use of medicines to bolster the viscera and external medicines attributed to Liu Juanzi 劉涓子 (ca. 370–450) for pediatric and other skin infections;

(6) recipes;

(7) *materia medica*, including versions of the *Newly Revised Materia Medica*, the Tang revision of Tao Hongjing's work (Liu 2021, 81-82), and *Shiliao bencao* 食療本草, a Tang book on dietetics;

(8) acumoxa treatments, theory, and prohibitions;

(9) various texts on magical or *yangsheng* methods;

(10) Buddhist and Daoist recipes; and

(11) random jottings of medical information on physicians, records, ailments, names and prices of medicines, and medical equipment.

Studies of select texts are included in collections edited by Vivienne Lo and Christopher Cullen (2005) and by Catherine Despeux (2010). Many manuscripts are scanned and available to the public in the IDP (International Dunhuang Project) database. Wang Shumin (2005) notes a number of new medical concepts: For the first time, the space between the temples is identified as a "host" (*zhu* 主) of the spiritual "essence" (*jing*) and "recognition, consciousness" (*shi* 識). Nine storage depots (*zang*) of *qi* include four belonging to the outer structure (*xing* 形) – corners of the head (temples), ears and eyes, mouth and teeth, chest and trunk; and five belonging to the spirit (*shen*) – heart, liver, spleen, lungs, and kidneys. Among the fragmentary acumoxa texts, the locations of points listed for treatment of specified conditions or for calibrating the *qi* in various viscera differ from those in medical canons and are often inconsistent among different Dunhuang manuscripts, suggesting that there were no fixed points even by the tenth century (Lo, 2005, 207–251; Lo, 2010, 239–284). The number and names of the points also vary. Some points or "openings" (*xue*) were specified as for *qi* and others for wind (for wind as a cause of insanity, see Chen Hsiu-fen, 2005). There were also multiple other spiritual or supernatural entities in the body that could affect acumoxa practice (this is particularly the case with regard to calendrical prohibitions; see Harper, 2005; Arrault, 2010).

Pulse-reading texts vary in their numbers of pulse types and which indicate a fatal condition or when to add drug therapy – generally differing from the canon *Maijing* (for pulse-reading with physiognomy; see Despeux, 2005; for pulse-reading, see Hsu, 2010). Manuscripts of *materia medica* and recipes record drug applications and therapies, such as one to treat acute heart pain with saltpeter and realgar (see Butler and Moffett, 2005; Despeux, 2010, 333–629; Engelhardt, 2010). Self-cultivation and sexual practices continued to be part of the healing literature (Lo & Cullen, 2005, 207–290).

Magical medicine, including Daoist, Buddhist, and popular practices, persisted (Strickmann, 2002). It was often transmitted as "secret instructions" (*jue* 決 for 訣), such as *Master Qing Wu's Secret Instructions on the Pulse* (*Qing Wuzi maijue* 青烏子脈決, P.3655) and *Wondrous Instructions on the Skill of Quiescent Breathing* (*Huxi jinggong miaojue* 呼吸靜功妙決, P.3810). Qing Wuzi (Master Blue Crow) is identified as the sixth-century master of *yin*-and-*yang* divination, Xiao Ji 蕭吉 (Ma Jixing, 1988, 92–93; Harper, 2010a, 39, 66–72). It is the last of three medical texts probably dating to the early Tang found on P.3655 that take up a total of ninety-seven columns of text. The first two are the *Illuminated Hall Treatise of the Five Viscera* (*Mingtang wuzang lun* 明堂五臟論) and *The Seven Superficial and Eight Deep Pulses in the Three Sectors* (*Qi biao ba li san bu mai* 七表八理三部脈). The text by Qing Wuzi appears on columns 64–79. It is essentially a version of the *Verses for Examining the Pulses of the Left and Right Wrists* (*Zuoyou shou zhenmai ge* 左右手診脈) preserved in the *Wang Shuhe mai jue* 王叔和脈訣 (also known simply as the *Maijue* by the Song period). It includes seven verses, all in heptasyllabic meter (*qiyan gejue* 七言歌訣) (for medieval phonetic reconstruction, see Baxter & Sargart, 2014). The first verse is an overview of pulse diagnostics:

> Left and right reveal the signs of the pulses in the four seasons (over the course of) 45 (pulse) movements during one full breath. If below the finger (of the physician pressing down) (the pulse) is urgent or full, there is Wind Toxin increasing the indicator of Heat. If below the finger, it is slow, deep, and thin, then a Cold ailment has overtaken the body along with Wind *qi*. In the case of a (demonically infected) stolen vessel, one typically asks about the Five Agents and in the case of dripping or blocked (vessels) there is no cure.

> 左右須候四時脈 (*meak*)，四十五動為一息 (*sik*)。
> 指下如法急緊洪 (*huwngH*)，兼有風毒加熱機 (*kjj*)。
> 指下遲遲脈沉細 (*sejH*)，冷病纏身並風氣 (*khjjH*)。
> 賊脈頻來問五行 (*haengH*)，屋漏陸門終不治 (*driH*)。

The next six verses on pulses (*mai ge* 脈歌) deal with the pulses in the *cun* 寸, *guan* 關, and *chi* 尺 positions on the left and right wrists as diagnostic criteria for the viscera: (1) the left wrist *cun* opening (*kou* 口) to the Heart (*xin*), (2) left wrist middle indicator (*zhongzhi* 中指) to the Liver sector (*gan bu*), (3) left wrist *chi hong* 尺中 to the Kidney sector (*shen bu*), (4) right wrist *cun kou* to the Lung sector (*fei bu*), (5) right wrist *zhongzhi* to the Spleen sector (*pi bu*), (6) right wrist *chi zhong* to the Gate of Life (*mingmen* 命門) (Ma Jixing, 1988, 93–96).

The second text, *Wondrous Instructions on the Skill of Quiescent Breathing*, a self-cultivation text, consists of sixteen columns of text possibly copied in the ninth century. The breath techniques focused on the circulation of blood and *qi* and on the fortifying of primordial *qi* (*yuanqi*). This involved regulating the emotions. Various Daoist techniques and spells boosted the cosmic *qi* in the body, allowing for revitalization and long life, if not total escape from mortality altogether.

Materia medica for strengthening the body also qualified as technical secrets. In another text known as *Buxing jue* 輔行決 (also called the *Secret Instructions for Assisting the Body, also called the Essential Methods for the Application of Drugs to the Viscera and Bowels* 輔行決臟腑用藥法要 by the physicians in China who preserved copies), longevity drugs were traced to Tao Hongjing (Ma Jixing, 1992, 115). In fact, the teachings, passed on by a "hermit" (*yinju* 隱居), draw from the Han period *Canonical Methods for Brews and Decoctions* (*Tangye jingfa* 湯液經法) and include fifty-six recipes and the "rules of reinforcing and reducing methods for the five viscera" (五臟補瀉法例), focusing on the correlation of drugs with the Five Agents and five flavors. It also includes the earliest remedies for infectious diseases (*tianxing* 天行). Many of the recipes continued to be handed down and appear in existing versions of the *Treatise on Cold Damage* and the *Treatise on the Essential Prescriptions of the Golden Casket* (Ma Jixing, 1992, 115–137; Wang & Barret, 2005). The "hermit" editor explained that the purpose of the text was to make sure that healers knew to go beyond simply supplementing or discharging (*bu xie* 補瀉) the perverse *qi* (*xie qi*) that had entered the body. Because the process of dealing with the evil *qi* also threatened the person's "spiritual essence" and *qi*, it was essential to bolster the *qi* of the five viscera with multiple doses of medicinal decoctions. Without this extra step, the viscera could become depleted and over time harmed to the point of risking death (Fruehauf & Dell'orfano, 2015: preface).

The Dunhuang materials reveal the range of medieval healing practices. They reflect the rise of court-sponsored medical canons but also the many materials left out of them. They reinforce the entwined nature of magical medicine with cosmic medicine but also show the persistence of drug experimentation and herbal decoctions.

4 Conclusion

Non-transmitted textual material – preserved on bones, bronzes, bamboo, silk, and paper – reflect ideas and treatments for maintaining human well-being that are not reflected in the transmitted medical canons. Yet, by the end of the Han, we can see the development of methods and concepts that will eventually coalesce in literati writings. Cosmic or *yinyang wuxing* medicine dealing with the perverse influences of environmental *qi* was intermixed with magical practices that addressed spirits and demons. A shift from simple external observation to inclusion of diagnostic methods of internal disorders occurred while symptom clusters also began to be defined as specific ailments. Manuscripts also reveal the diversity of practices preserved and changed over time by physicians and healers of different social statuses and locales.

Archaic Graphs

1 ⬚ Shang oracle bone graph for 蚩 > 毒 *du* "toxin"

2 ⬚ ⬚ ⬚ Shang oracle bone graphs for 疾 *ji* "affliction"

3 ⬚ ⬚ Early Zhou graphs for 殷 Yin, the Zhou name for the Shang people. Also a rare Shang word possibly for a medical procedure.

4 ⬚ Huayuanzhuang bone graph for some type of healing.

5 ⬚ ⬚ Shang oracle bone graphs for 禦 *yu* "drive away, ward off, exorcise"

Bibliography

Allan, Sarah. 1991. *The Shape of the Turtle: Myth, Art, and Cosmos in Early China*. Albany: State University of New York.

Allan, Sarah. 2015. "'When Red Pigeons Gathered on Tang's House': A Warring States Period Tale of Shamanic Possession and Building Construction Set at the Turn of the Xia and Shang Dynasties." *Journal of the Royal Asiatic Society* 25.3: 419–438.

Arrault, Alain. 2010. "Activités médicales et methods héméologiques dans les calendriers de Dunhuang du IXe au Xe siècle: esprit humain (*renshen*) et esprit du jour (*riyou*)." In Catherine Despeux, ed. *Médecine, religion et société dans la Chine médiévale: Les manuscrits médicaux de Dunhuang et de Turfan*, Vol. 1. Paris: Collège de France, Institut des Hautes Études Chinoises, 285–332.

Barbieri-Low, Anthony J. & Robin D. S. Yates. 2015. *Law, State, and Society in Early Imperial China: A Study with Critical Edition and Translation of the Legal Texts from Zhangjiashan Tomb No. 247*. 2 vols. Leiden: Brill.

Baxter, William H. & Laurent Sagart. 2014. *Old Chinese: A New Reconstruction*. Oxford: Oxford University Press.

Beijing daxue chutu wenxian yanjiusuo 北京大學出土文獻研究所 [Beijing University Excavated Text Research Institute], ed. 2013. *Beijing daxue cang Qin dai jiandushuji xuancui* 北京大學藏秦代簡牘書迹選粹 [*Selections of Qin Bamboo and Wooden Textual Traces Preserved by Beijing University*]. Beijing: Renmin yishu.

Bian, He. 2020. *Know Your Remedies: Pharmacy and Culture in Early Modern China*. Princeton, NJ: Princeton University Press.

Brindley, Erica F. 2013. "The Cosmos As Creative Mind: Spontaneous Arising, Generating, and Creating in the *Heng Xian*." *Dao: A Journal of Comparative Philosophy* 12.2: 189–206.

Brown, Miranda. 2015. *The Art of Medicine in Early China: The Ancient and Medieval Origins of a Modern Archive*. Cambridge: Cambridge University Press.

Buell, Paul & Eugene N. Anderson. 2021. *Arabic Medicine in China: Tradition, Innovation, and Change*. Leiden: Brill.

Butler, Anthony & John Moffet. "A Treatment for Cardiovascular Dysfunction in a Dunhuang Medical Manuscript." In Vivienne Lo & Christopher Cullen, eds. *Medieval Chinese Medicine: The Dunhuang Medical Manuscripts*. London: Routledge, 363–368.

Caboara, Marco. 2016. "Drought, Omens and the Body Politic: Debates between Rulers and Ministers in the Shanghai Museum Manuscript 'Jian da wang po han.'" *Bulletin of the Jao Tsung-I Academy of Sinology* 饒宗頤國學院院刊 2016.3: 47–75.

Cao Feng 曹峰. 2012. "*Hengxian* de qi lun – yizhong xin de wanwu shengcheng dongli moshi" "恆先" 的氣論 – 一種新的萬物生成動力模式 [The Theory of *qi* in the *Hengxian*: A Dynamic New Pattern for the Creation of All Things]. *Zhongguo zhexue* 中國哲學 [*Chinese Philosophy*] 2012.5: 42–51.

Cao Feng. 2019. "Qinghua jian *Tang zai Chimen* yizhu" 清華簡 《湯在啻門》譯注. In Li Xueqin 李學勤, Ai Lan 艾蘭, Lü Dekai 呂德凱 eds. 2019. *Qinghua daxue cang Zhangguo zhujian (wu)* Guoji xueshu yantaohui lunwenji 《清華大學藏戰國竹簡(伍)》國際學術研討會論文集 [Collected Essays from the International Seminar on Vol. 5 of the *Warring States Bamboo Slips Stored at Qinghua University*]. *Qinghua jian yanjiu* 清華簡研究 [*Qinghua Bamboo Slip Research*] 3. Shanghai: Zhongxi, 108–143.

Cao Jianguo 曹建國. 2020. "Cong Liubo liu *Jing Gong nüe* kan *Yanzi* zaoqi wenben xingtai" 從上博六《景公瘧》看《晏子》早期文本形態 [Examining the Early Format of *Yanzi* Text from the *Jing Gong Lüe* in Shanghai Museum Volume 6]. *Beijing shehui kexue* 北京社會科學 [*Beijing Social Science*] 2020.5: 37–47.

Chang, Tsung-tung. 1970. *Der Kult der Shang-dynastie im Spiegel der Orakelinschriften: Eine paläographische Studie zur religion im archaischen China*. Wiesbaden: Otto Harrassowitz.

Chen Guangyu 陳光宇, Song Zhenhao 宋鎮豪, Liu Yuan 劉源, & An Maxiu 安馬修 (Matt Anderson), eds. 2017. *Shangdai jiagu Zhong-ying duben* 商代甲骨中英讀本 *Reading of Shang Inscriptions*. Shanghai: Renmin.

Chen Hsiu-fen. "Wind Malady As Madness in Medieval China: Some Threads from the Dunhuang Medical Manuscript." In Vivienne Lo & Christopher Cullen, eds. *Medieval Chinese Medicine: The Dunhuang Medical Manuscripts*. London: Routledge, 345–362.

Chen Hui 陳慧 (Shirley Chan). 2019. "Shenti yu zhi guo: shidu Qinghua jian *Tang zai Chimen* jian lun 'ji'" 身體與治國—試讀清華簡《湯在啻門》兼論 "疾" [Body and Healing the State: Pondering the Qinghua Bamboo Text *Tang zai Chimen* and the Term *ji*]. In Li Xueqin 李學勤, Ai Lan 艾蘭, Lü Dekai 呂德凱 eds. 2019. *Qinghua daxue cang Zhangguo zhujian (wu)* Guoji xueshu yantaohui lunwenji 《清華大學藏戰國竹簡(伍)》國際學術研討會論文集 [Collected Essays from the International Seminar on Vol. 5 of the *Warring States Bamboo Slips Stored at Qinghua*

University]. *Qinghua jian yanjiu* 清華簡研究 [*Qinghua Bamboo Slip Research*] 3. Shanghai: Zhongxi, 171–182.

Chen Shihui 陳世輝. 1963. "Yin ren jibin bukao" 殷人疾病補考 [Addendum to Illnesses of the Yin People]. *Zhonghua wenshi luncong* 中華文史論叢 [*Essays on Chinese Literature and History*] Vol. 4. Shanghai: Zhonghua, 138.

Chen Wei 陳偉. 2005. "Du Shashi Zhoujiatai Qin jian zhaji" 讀沙市周家臺秦簡札記 [Notes on the Qin Bamboo Strips from the Sha City Zhoujiatai Tomb]. *Jianbo* [*Bamboo and Silk*], November 2. http://m.bsm.org.cn/?qinjian/4284.html (accessed March 3, 2023).

Chen Wei. 2009. *Chudi chutu Zhanguo jiance (shisi zhong)* 楚地出土戰國簡冊 (十四種) [*Fourteen Types of Warring States Bamboo Texts Excavated from the Chu Region*]. Beijing: Jingji kexue.

Chen Wei. 2012. *Liye Qin Jiandu jiaoyi* 里耶秦簡牘校釋 [*Exegeses of Qin Bamboo and Wooden Texts from Liye*], Vol. 1. Wuhan: Wuhan University Press.

Chen Wei. In press. "Transcription Notes on the Tsinghua Bamboo Text *The Heart Is Called the Center*." In Constance A. Cook, Christopher Foster, & Susan Blader, eds., *Metaphor and Meaning: Thinking About Early China with Sarah Allan*. Albany: State University of New York.

Cook, Constance A. 2006. *Death in Ancient China: The Tale of One Man's Journey*. Leiden: Brill.

Cook, Constance A. 2013a. "The Ambiguity of Text, Birth, and Nature." *Dao: A Journal of Comparative Philosophy* 12.2: 161–178.

Cook, Constance A. 2013b. "The Pre-Han Period." In T. J. Hinrichs & Linda L. Barnes, eds., *Chinese Medicine and Healing: An Illustrated History*. Cambridge, MA: Belknap Press, 5–29.

Cook, Constance A. 2016. "A Fatal Case of Gu 蠱 Poisoning in the Fourth Century BC?" *East Asian Science, Technology, and Medicine* 44: 61–122.

Cook, Constance A. 2017. *Ancestors, Kings, and the Dao*. Cambridge, MA: Harvard Asia Center.

Cook, Constance A. "Contextualizing 'Becoming a Complete Person' in the *Tang zai Chimen*." In Li Xueqin 李學勤, Ai Lan 艾蘭, Lü Dekai 呂德凱 eds. 2019. *Qinghua daxue cang Zhangguo zhujian (wu)* Guoji xueshu yantaohui lunwenji 《清華大學藏戰國竹簡(伍)》國際學術研討會論文集 [Collected Essays from the International Seminar on Vol. 5 of the *Warring States Bamboo Slips Stored at Qinghua University*]. *Qinghua jian yanjiu* 清華簡研究 [*Qinghua Bamboo Slip Research*] 3. Shanghai: Zhongxi, 183–193.

Cook, Constance A. 2021. "Qi." *Encyclopedia of Ancient History: Asia and Africa*. Wiley Online Library. https://doi.org/10.1002/9781119399919.eahaa00778.

Cook, Constance A. In press. "Exorcism and the Spirit Turtle." In Constance A. Cook, Christopher Foster, & Susan Blader, eds., *Metaphor and Meaning: Thinking About Early China with Sarah Allan*. Albany: State University of New York.

Cook, Constance A., Christopher Foster, & Susan Blader, eds. In press. *Metaphor and Meaning: Thinking About Early China with Sarah Allan*. Albany: State University of New York.

Cook, Constance A. & Xinhui Luo. 2017. *Birth in Ancient China: A Study of Metaphor and Cultural Identity in Pre-imperial China*. Albany: State University of New York.

Cook, Constance A. & Zhao Lu. 2017. *Stalk Images: A Newly Discovered Alternative to the* I-ching. Oxford: Oxford University Press.

Despeux, Catherine. 2001. "The System of Five Circulatory Phases and the Six Seasonal Influences (*wuyun liuqi*): A Source of Innovation in Medicine under the Song." In Elisabeth Hsu, ed., *Innovation in Chinese Medicine*. Cambridge: Cambridge University Press, 121–165.

Despeux, Catherine. 2005. "From Prognosis to Diagnosis of Illness in Tang China: Comparison of the Dunhuang Manuscript P. 3390 and Medical Sources." In Vivienne Lo & Christopher Cullen, eds., *Medieval Chinese Medicine: The Dunhuang Medical Manuscripts*. London: Routledge, 176–206.

Despeux, Catherine. 2007. "Âmes et animation du corps: La notion de shen dans la médecine chinoise antique," *Extrême-Orient, Extrême-Occident* 29, *De l'esprit aux exprits. Enquête sur la notion de shen. Of Self and Spirits: Exploring Shen in China*, 71–94.

Despeux, Catherine. 2010. "Les recettes médicamenteuses de Dunhuang." In Catherine Despeux, ed. *Médecine, religion et société dans la Chine médiévale: Les manuscrits médicaux de Dunhuang et de Turfan*, Vol. 1. Paris: Collège de France, Institut des Hautes Études Chinoises, 333–629.

Despeux, Catherine, ed. 2010. *Médecine, religion et société dans la Chine médiévale: Les manuscrits médicaux de Dunhuang et de Turfan*. 3 vols. Paris: Collège de France, Institut des Hautes Études Chinoises.

Dotson, Brandon, Constance A. Cook, & Zhao Lu. 2021. *Dice and Gods on the Silk Road: Chinese Buddhist Dice Divination in Transcultural Context*. Prognostication in History 7. Leiden: Brill.

Du Feng 杜鋒. 2014a. "Qinghua jian *Chi hu zhi ji Tang wu* yu wuyi jiaohe" 清華簡《赤鵠之集湯屋》與巫醫校合 [Collation of Ideas Concerning Shaman Doctors and the Qinghua Bamboo Text *Chihe zhi ji Tang wu*. *Shiliao yanjiu* 史料研究 [*Research into Historical Materials*] 2014.2: 4–5.

Du Feng. 2014b. "Laoguanshan yijian zhong de 'pie xi' yu Bian Que minghao" 老官山醫簡中的"敝昔"與扁鵲名號 [Bian Que and the Name Pie Xi in the Laoguanshan Bamboo Medical Texts]. *Mingzuo xinshang* 名作欣賞 [*Appreciation of Masterpieces*] 2014.8: 15–16.

Du Zhengsheng 杜正勝. 2005. *Cong meishou dao changsheng – yiliao wenhua yu Zhongguo gudai shengmingguan.* 從眉壽到長生－醫療文化與中國古代生命觀 [*From* meishou *to* Changsheng*: The Culture of Healing and View on Life in Ancient China*]. Taipei: Sanmin.

Engelhardt, Ute. 2001. "Dietetics in Tang China and the First Extant Work of *Materia dietetica.*" In Elisabeth Hsu, ed., *Innovation in Chinese Medicine.* Cambridge: Cambridge University Press, 173–191.

Engelhardt, Ute. 2010. "Pharmacopées de Dunhuang et de Turfan." In Catherine Despeux, ed. *Médecine, religion et société dans la Chine médiévale: Les manuscrits médicaux de Dunhuang et de Turfan*, Vol. 1. Paris: Collège de France, Institut des Hautes Études Chinoises, 185–237.

Fan Ka-wai. 2013. "The Period of Division and the Tang Period." In T. J. Hinrichs & Linda L. Barnes, eds., *Chinese Medicine and Healing: An Illustrated History.* Cambridge, MA: Belknap Press, 65–96.

Fan Yuzhou 范毓周. 1998. "'Yin ren jibing bukao' bianzheng" "殷人疾病補考"辨證 [Debating 'Addendum on Illnesses of the Yin People']. *Dongnan wenhua* 東南文化 [*Southwestern Culture*] 1998.3: 99.

Fang Yong 方勇 & Hou Na 侯娜. 2015. "Du Zhoujiatai Qin jian yifang zhaji (erce)" 讀周家台秦簡醫方札記(二則) [Two Notes on the Qin Bamboo Medical Recipes from Zhoujiatai]. *Ludong daxue xuebao* 魯東大學學報 [*Ludong University Journal*] 2015.3: 52–54.

Fang Yong & Hu Junyi 胡润怡. 2015. "Du Qin yifang jian zhaji erze" 讀秦醫方簡札記二則. *Changchun shifan daxue xuebao* 長春師範大學學報 2015.7: 69–71.

Feng Yicheng 風儀誠 (Olivier Venture). 2019 "Du Qinghuajian *Yin Gaozong wen yu sanshou, Tang chuyu Tangqiu, Tang zai Chimen* sanpien zhaji" 讀清華簡《殷高宗問於三壽》《湯處於湯丘》《湯在啻門》三篇札記 [Notes on the Three Qinghua Bamboo Texts *Yin Gaozong wen yu sanshou, Tang chuyu Tangqiu*, and *Tang zai Chimen*]. In Li Xueqin 李學勤, Ai Lan 艾蘭, Lü Dekai 呂德凱 eds. *Qinghua daxue cang Zhangguo zhujian (wu)* Guoji xueshu yantaohui lunwenji 《清華大學藏戰國竹簡(伍)》國際學術研討會論文集 [Collected Essays from the International Seminar on Vol. 5 of the *Warring States Bamboo Slips Stored at Qinghua University*]. *Qinghua jian yanjiu* 清華簡研究 [*Qinghua Bamboo Slip Research*] 3. Shanghai: Zhongxi, 55–77.

Fruehauf, Heiner & Michael Dell'orfano. 2015. Fuxing Jue and Tangye Jing Translation Project. *Classical Chinese Medicine*. https://classicalchineseme dicine.org/articles/member-articles/ (accessed March 17, 2023).

Furth, Charlotte. 1999. *A Flourishing Yin: Gender in China's Medical History, 960–1665*. Berkeley: University of California Press.

Gansusheng wenwu kaogu yanjiusuo 甘肅省文物考古研究所 [Gansu Province Relics and Archaeological Research Institute], ed. 2009. *Tianshui Fangmatan Qin jian* 天水放馬灘秦簡 [*The Qin Bamboo Slips of Fangmatan in Tianshui*]. Beijing: Zhonghua.

Guo Lihua 郭梨華 (Kuo Li-hua). 2019 "Qinghua jian (wu) guanyu 'wei' zhi zhexue tanjiu" 清華簡(伍)關於"味"之哲學探究 [A Philosophical Investigation of the Term *wei* (flavor) in Volume 5 of the Qinghua University Bamboo Slips]. In Li Xueqin 李學勤, Ai Lan 艾蘭, Lü Dekai 呂德凱 eds. *Qinghua daxue cang Zhangguo zhujian (wu)* Guoji xueshu yantaohui lunwenji 《清華大學藏戰國竹簡(伍)》國際學術研討會論文集 [Collected Essays from the International Seminar on Vol. 5 of the *Warring States Bamboo Slips Stored at Qinghua University*]. *Qinghua jian yanjiu* 清華簡研究 [*Qinghua Bamboo Slip Research*] 3. Shanghai: Zhongxi, 222–236.

Hanson, Marta E. 2011. *Speaking of Epidemics in Chinese Medicine: Disease and the Geographic Imagination in Late Imperial China*. Needham Research Institute Series. London: Routledge.

Hanson, Marta E. 2020. "From Under the Elbow to Pointing to the Palm: Chinese Metaphors for Learning Medicine by the Book (Fourth–Fourteenth Centuries)." *BJHS Themes* 5: 75–92.

Harper, Donald J. 1985. "A Chinese Demonography of the Third Century B.C." *Harvard Journal of Asiatic Studies* 45: 459–498.

Harper, Donald J. 1990. "The Conception of Illness in Early Chinese Medicine, As Documented in Newly Discovered 3rd and 2nd Century B.C. Manuscripts (Part I)." *Sudhoffs Archiv* 74.2: 210–235.

Harper, Donald J. 1998. *Early Chinese Medical Literature: The Mawangdui Medical Manuscripts*. London: Kegan Paul International.

Harper, Donald J. 1999a. "Warring States: Natural Philosophy and Occult Thought." In M. Loewe & E. L. Shaughnessy, eds. *The Cambridge History of Ancient China: From the Origins of Civilization to 221 BC*. Cambridge: Cambridge University Press, 813–884.

Harper, Donald J. 1999b. "Physicians and Diviners: The Relation of Divination to the Medicine of the Huangdi neijing (Inner Canon of the Yellow Thearch)." *Divination et rationalité en Chine ancienne*. No. 21: *Extrême-Orient Extrême-Occident*: 91–110.

Harper, Donald J. 2001. "Iatromancy, Diagnosis, and Prognosis in Early Chinese Medicine." In Elisabeth Hsu, ed., *Innovation in Chinese Medicine*. Cambridge: Cambridge University Press, 99–120.

Harper, Donald J. 2005. "Dunhuang Iatromantic Manuscripts P. 2856 R° and P. 2675 V°." In Vivienne Lo & Christopher Cullen, eds., *Medieval Chinese Medicine: The Dunhuang Medical Manuscripts*. London: Routledge, 134–164.

Harper, Donald J. 2010a. "The Textual Form of Knowledge: Occult Miscellanies in Ancient and Medieval Chinese Manuscripts, Fourth Century B.C. to Tenth Century A.D." In Florence Bretelle-Esteblet, ed. *Looking at It from Asia: The Processes That Shaped the Sources of History of Science*. Dordrecht: Springer, 37–80.

Harper, Donald J. 2010b. "Précis de connaissance médicale. Le *Shanghan lun* 傷寒論 (Traité des atteintes par le Froid) et le *Wuzang lun* 五藏論 (Traité des cinq vixcères)." In Catherine Despeux, ed. *Médecine, religion et société dans la Chine médiévale: Les manuscrits médicaux de Dunhuang et de Turfan*, Vol. 1. Paris: Collège de France, Institut des Hautes Études Chinoises, 65–106.

Harper, Donald & Marc Kalinowski, eds. 2017. *Books of Fate and Popular Culture in Early China: The Daybook Manuscripts of the Warring States, Qin, and Han*. Handbook of Oriental Studies (Handbuch der Orientalistik): Section 4 China Series. Leiden: Brill.

Hendrischke, Barbara. 2006. *"The Scripture on Great Peace" The* Taiping Jing *and the Beginnings of Daoism*. Berkeley: University of California Press.

Hinrichs, T. J. & Linda L. Barnes, eds. 2013. *Chinese Medicine and Healing: An Illustrated History*. Cambridge, MA: Belknap Press of Harvard University.

Hou Naifeng 侯乃峰. 2005. "Qin Yin dao bing yuban mingwen jishi" 秦駰禱病玉版銘文集釋, *Wenbo*文博 2005.6: 69–75.

Hsu, Elisabeth, ed. 2001. *Innovation in Chinese Medicine*. Cambridge: Cambridge University Press.

Hsu, Elisabeth. 2007. "The Experience of Wind in Early and Medieval Chinese Medicine." *The Journal of the Royal Anthropological Institute* 13: S117–S134.

Hsu, Elisabeth. 2008–9. "Outward Form (*xing* 形) and Inward Qi: The 'Sentimental Body' in Early Chinese Medicine." *Early China* 32: 103–124.

Hsu, Elisabeth. 2010a. *Pulse Diagnosis in Early Chinese Medicine: The Telling Touch*. Cambridge: Cambridge University Press.

Hsu, Elisabeth. 2010b. "Le diagnostic du pouls dans la Chine médiévale d'après les manuscrits de Dunhuang." In Catherine Despeux, ed. *Médecine, religion et société dans la Chine médiévale: Les manuscrits médicaux de Dunhuang et de Turfan*, Vol. 1. Paris: Collège de France, Institut des Hautes Études Chinoises, 107–184.

Hu Houxuan 胡厚宣. 1942. "Yin ren jibing kao" 殷人疾病考 [Examination of the Illnesses of the People of Yin]. *Jiagu xue Shang shi luncong* 甲骨學商史論叢 [*Essays on Oracle Bone Studies and Shang History*]. Chengdu: Qi Lu daxue guxue yanjiusuo.

Hu Houxuan. 1984. "Lun Yin ren zhiliao jibing zhi fangfa" 論殷人治療疾病之方法 [The Yin People's Methods for Healing Illness]. *Zhongyuan wenwu* 中原文物 [*Central Plains Relics*] 1984.4: 27–30.

Huang Dekun 黃德寬. 2013. "Qinghua jian *Chihe zhi ji Tang zhi wu* yu Xian Qin 'xiaoshuo' – lüeshuo Qinghua jian dui Xian Qin wenxue yanjiu de jiazhi" 清華簡《赤鵠之集湯之屋》與先秦"小說"–略說清華簡對先秦文學研究的價值 [Qinghua Bamboo *Chihe zhi ji Tang zhi wu* and Pre-Qin Fiction: Notes on the Value of the Qinghua Bamboo Texts to the Study of Pre-Qin Literature]. *Fudan xuebao* 復旦學報 [*Fudan Academic Journal*] 2013.4: 81–86.

Huang Guanyun 黃冠雲 (Huan Kuan-yun). 2019 "Shuo *Tang zai Chimen* lun 'qi' yi jie wenzi" 說《湯在啻門》論"氣"一節文字 [The Word *qi* in the *Tang zai Chimen*]. In Li Xueqin 李學勤, Ai Lan 艾蘭, Lü Dekai 呂德凱 eds. *Qinghua daxue cang Zhangguo zhujian (wu)* Guoji xueshu yantaohui lunwenji《清華大學藏戰國竹簡(伍)》國際學術研討會論文集 [Collected Essays from the International Seminar on Vol. 5 of the *Warring States Bamboo Slips Stored at Qinghua University*]. *Qinghua jian yanjiu* 清華簡研究 [*Qinghua Bamboo Slip Research*] 3. Shanghai: Zhongxi, 159–170.

Huang Tianshu 黃天樹. 2006. *Guwenzi lunji* 古文字論集 [*Collected Essays on Paleography*]. Beijing: Xueyuan.

Huang-fu Mi (215–282). 1994. *The Systematic Classic of Acupuncture and Moxibustion*. Translation of the *Jia Yi Jing* by Yang Shou-zhong & Charles Chace, 16th ed. Portland, OR: Black Poppy Press, 2020.

Hubeisheng Jingzhoushi Zhouliang yuqiao yizhi bowuguan 湖北省荊州市周梁玉橋遺址博物館 [Hubei Provincial Jingzhou City Museum of the Zhouliang yuqiao Site], ed. 2001. *Guanju Qin Han mu jiandu* 關沮秦漢墓簡牘 [*Bamboo and Wood Slips from Qin and Han Tombs in Guanzhu*]. Beijing: Zhonghua.

Hubeisheng wenwu kaogu yanjiusuo 湖北省文物考古研究所 [Hubei Provincial Relic and Archeology Research Institute]. 1996. *Jiangling Wangshan Shazhong Chu mu* 江陵望山沙冢楚墓 [*Chu Tombs at Shazhong, Wangshan, Jiangling*]. Beijing: Wenwu.

Hubeisheng wenwu kaogu yanjiusuo & Beijing daxue zhongwenxi 北京大學中文系 [Beijing University Chinese Department], eds. 1999. *Jiudian Chu jian* 九店楚簡 [*Chu Bamboo Slips at Jiudian*]. Beijing: Zhonghua.

Hunter, Michael. 2018. "The 'Yiwen zhi' 藝文志 (Treatise on Arts and Letters) Bibliography in Its Own Context." *Journal of the American Oriental Society* 138.4: 763–780.

Jingmenshi bowuguan 荊門市博物館 [Jingmen City Museum].1998. *Guodian Chu mu zhujian* 郭店楚墓竹簡 [*Bamboo Slips from a Chu Tomb in Guodian*]. Beijing: Wenwu.

Ke Heli 柯鶴立 (Constance A. Cook) & Cai Lili 蔡麗利. 2021. "Guanyu 'xin' zai Han yiqian chutu wenxian zhong suo biaoshi de shenti buwei ji qi neihan bianhua de yanjiu" 關於"心"在漢以前出土文獻中所表示的身體部位及其內涵變化的研究 [Changes in the Physical Location of the *xin* (heart) According to Pre-Han Excavated Texts." In Qinghua Daxue chutu wenxian yanjiu yu baohu zhongxin 清華大學出土文獻研究與保護中心 [Qinghua University Center for Research and Preservation of Excavated Text] ed., *Banbu xueshu shi, yiwei Li xiansheng – Li Xueqin xiansheng xueshu chengjiu yu xueshu sixiang guoji yantaohui lun wenji* 半部學術史,一位李先生 – 李學勤先生學術成就與學術思想國際研討會論文集 [*A Partial History of Mr Li: Collected Essays from the International Seminar in Honor of Academic Accomplishments and Thought of Mr. Li Xueqin*]. Shanghai: Zhongxi, 883–894.

Ke Heli. 2022. 周代 "明心":一種統治工具 [A Zhou Tool for Enlightenment]. In Li Feng 李峰 & Shi Jingsong 施勁松, eds., *Zhang Changshou, Cheng Gongrou jinian wenji* 張長壽、陳公柔先生紀念文集 [*Collected Essays in Memory of Zhang Changshou and Chen Gongrou*]. Beijing: Chinese Academy of Social Sciences, Institute for Archaeology, 489–502.

Keegan, David J. 1988. "The *Huang-ti nei-ching*: The Structure of the Compilation; The Significance of the Structure." PhD dissertation, University of California, Berkeley .

Keightley, David N. 2000. *The Ancestral Landscape: Time, Space, and Community in Late Shang China (ca. 1200–1045 B.C.)*. China Research Monograph 53. Institute of East Asian Studies. Berkeley: University of California Press.

Keightley, David N. 2012. *Working for His Majesty: Research Notes on Labor Mobilization in Late Shang China (ca.1200–1045 B.C.), As Seen in the Oracle-Bone Inscriptions, with Particular Attention to Handicraft Industries, Agriculture, Warfare, Hunting, Construction, and the Shang's Legacies*. China Research Monograph 67. Institute of East Asian Studies. Berkeley: University of California Press.

Knoblock John. 1988. *Xunzi: A Translation and Study of the Complete Works*. 3 vols. Stanford, CA: Stanford University Press.

Lan Riyong 藍日勇. 1993. "Guangxi Guixian Han mu chutu yinzhen de yanjiu" 廣西貴縣漢墓出土銀針的研究 [A Study of the Silver Needles Excavated from a Han Tomb in Guixian, Guangxi]. *Nanfang wenwu* 南方文物 [*Southern Relics*] 1993.3: 64–66.

Lewis, Mark Edward. 2006a. *The Construction of Space in Early China*. Albany: State University of New York Press.

Lewis, Mark Edward. 2006b. *Flood Myths of Early China*. Albany: State University of New York Press.

Li Jianmin 李建民. 2000. *Sisheng zhi yu: Zhou Qin Han maixue zhi yuanliu* 死生之域:周秦漢脈學之源流 [*The Realm of Life and Death: The Origins of Vessel Theory in the Zhou, Qin, and Han Eras*]. Taipei: Zhongguo yuan-jiuyuan lishi yuyan yanjiusuo.

Li Jianmin. 2007. *Faxian gu mai: Zhongguo gudian yixue yu shushu shenti guan* 發現古脈:中國古典醫學與數術身體觀 [*Discovering Ancient Vessels: Classic Chinese Medicine and Technical Arts Theories of the Body*]. Beijing: Shehui kexue wenxian.

Li Ling 李零. 2000. *Zhongguo fangshu kao* 中國方術考 [*A Study of Chinese Magical Arts*]. Beijing: Dongfang.

Li Ling. 2006. *Zhongguo fangshu xukao* 中國方術續考 [*Further Studies of Chinese Magical Arts*]. Beijing: Zhonghua.

Li, Wai-yee. 2007. *The Readability of the Past in Early Chinese Historiography*. Cambridge, MA: Harvard University Asia Center.

Li Xueqin 李學勤, ed. 2013. *Qinghua daxue cang Zhanguo zhujian* 清華大學藏戰國竹簡 [*Warring States Bamboo Slips Stored at Qinghua University*]. Vol. 4. Shanghai: Zhongxi.

Li Xueqin 李學勤, Ai Lan 艾蘭, Lü Dekai 呂德凱 eds. 2019. *Qinghua daxue cang Zhangguo zhujian (wu)* Guoji xueshu yantaohui lunwenji 《清華大學藏戰國竹簡(伍)》國際學術研討會論文集 [Collected Essays from the International Seminar on Vol. 5 of the *Warring States Bamboo Slips Stored at Qinghua University*]. *Qinghua jian yanjiu* 清華簡研究 [*Qinghua Bamboo Slip Research*] 3. Shanghai: Zhongxi.

Lin Qianliang 林乾良. 2014. "Lun jiaguwen 'ji' zi" 論甲骨文"疾"字 [The Graph for *ji* in Oracle Bone Script]. *Zhongyi yao wenhua* 中醫藥文化 [*The Culture of Chinese Medicines*] 2014.1: 41–44.

Lin Zhenbang 林振邦. 2019. "Xian Qin Liang Han jianbo yishu de jibingguan yanjiu" 先秦兩漢簡帛醫書的疾病觀研究 [Study on the Concept of Illness in Pre-Qin and Han Bamboo and Silk Medical Texts]. Beijing Zhongyiyao daxue 北京中醫藥大學 PhD dissertation, Beijing University of Chinese Medicine.

Liu Jie 劉杰 & Yuan Jun 袁峻, 1998. *Zhongguo bagua yixue* 中國八卦醫學 [*Trigram Medicine in China*]. Qingdao: Xinhua.

Liu Lexian 劉樂賢. 1995. "Shuihudi Qin jian rishu 're zi pian' yanjiu" 睡虎地 秦簡日書 '人字篇' 研究 [The "Diagrams of the Human Figure" in Shuihudi Qin Era Bamboo Daybooks]. *Jiang Han kaogu* 江漢考古 [*Jiang-Han Archaeology*] 1995.1: 58–61, 82–3.

Liu Xinfang 劉信芳, comp. 2011. *Chu jianbo tongjia huishi* 楚簡帛通假匯釋 [*Interpreting Loan Words in Chu Bamboo and Silk Texts*]. Beijing: Gaodeng jiaoyu.

Liu, Yan. 2021. *Healing with Poisons: Potent Medicines in Medieval China*. Seattle: University of Washington.

Lo, Vivienne. 1999. "Tracking the Pain: *Jue* and the Formation of a Theory of Circulating *qi* through the Channels." *Sudhoffs Archiv* 83.2: 191–210.

Lo, Vivienne. 2000. "Crossing the Neiguan 'Inner Pass': A *nei/wai* 'Inner/ Outer' Distinction in Early Chinese Medicine." *East Asia Science Technology and Medicine* 17: 15–65.

Lo, Vivienne. 2001. "*Huangdi Hama jing* (Yellow Emperor's Toad Canon)." *Asia Major* 14.2: 61–99.

Lo, Vivienne. 2002a. "Lithic Therapy in Early China." In P. A. Baker & G. Carr, eds., *Practitioners, Practices and Patients: New Approaches to Medical Archaeology and Anthropology*. Oxford: Oxbow Books, 195–220.

Lo, Vivienne. 2002b. "Spirit of Stone: Technical Considerations in the Treatment of the Jade Body." *Bulletin of the School of Oriental and African Studies* 65.1: 99–128.

Lo, Vivienne. 2005. "Quick and Easy Chinese Medicine: the Dunhuang Moxibustion Charts." In Vivienne Lo & Christopher Cullen, eds. *Medieval Chinese Medicine: The Dunhuang Medical Manuscripts*. London: Routledge, 227–251.

Lo, Vivienne. 2010. "Manuscrits de Dunhuang et de Khotan sur la moxibustion." In Catherine Despeux, ed. *Médecine, religion et société dans la Chine médiévale: Les manuscrits médicaux de Dunhuang et de Turfan*, Vol. 1. Paris: Collège de France, Institut des Hautes Études Chinoises, 239–284.

Lo, Vivienne. 2013. "The Han Period." In T. J. Hinrichs & Linda L. Barnes, eds., *Chinese Medicine and Healing: An Illustrated History*. Cambridge, MA: Belknap Press, 31–64.

Lo, Vivienne. 2014. *How to do the Gibbon Walk: a Translation of the Pulling Book (ca 186 BCE)*. Cambridge, UK: Needham Research Institute Working Papers 3. https://www.nri.org.uk/yinshu.pdf.

Lo, Vivienne. 2018a. "Medicine and Healing in Han China." In Alexander Jones, ed. *The Cambridge History of Science*. Vol. 1. Cambridge, UK: Cambridge University, 574–594.

Lo, Vivienne. 2018b. "Imagining Practice: Sense and Sensuality in Early Chinese Medical Illustration." In Lo & Barratt et al, eds. 69–88.

Lo, Vivienne & Penelope Barrett, eds. 2018. *Imagining Chinese Medicine*. Leiden: Brill.

Lo, Vivienne & Christopher Cullen, eds. 2005. *Medieval Chinese Medicine: The Dunhuang Medical Manuscripts*. London: Routledge.

Lo, Vivienne & Gu Man. In press. "Water As Homology in the Construction of Classical Chinese Medicine." In Constance A. Cook, Christopher Foster, & Susan Blader, eds. *Metaphor and Meaning: Thinking About Early China with Sarah Allan*. Albany: State University of New York Press.

Lo, Vivienne & He Zhiguo 何志國. 1996. "The Channels: A preliminary examination of a Lacquered Figurine from the Western Han Period." *Early China* 21, 81–123.

Lo, Vivienne & Li Jianmin. 2007. "Manuscripts, Received Texts, and the Healing Arts." In Michael Nylan & Michael Loewe, eds. *China's Early Empires: A Re-Appraisal*. Cambridge, UK: Cambridge University, 367–397.

Lo, Vivienne & Michael Stanley-Baker with Dolly Yang. 2022. *Routledge Handbook of Chinese Medicine*. New York: Routledge.

Lloyd, Geoffrey & Nathan Sivin. 2002. *The Way and the Word: Science and Medicine in Early China and Greece*. New Haven, CT: Yale University Press.

Ma Chengyuan 馬承源, ed. 2001–12. *Shanghai bowuguan cang Zhanguo Chu zhujian* 上海博物館藏戰國楚竹簡 [*Chu Bamboo Slips of the Warring States Era Stored in the Shanghai Museum*]. Vols. 1–9. Shanghai: Shanghai guji.

Ma Jixing 馬繼興. 1988. *Dunhuang guyiji kaoshi* 敦煌古醫籍考 [*Study of Dunhuang Ancient Medical Records*]. Nanchang: Jiangxi kexue jishu.

Ma Jixing. 1992. *Mawangdui guyishu kaoshi* 馬王堆古醫書考釋 [*Interpretation of the Mawangdui Ancient Medical Books*]. Hunan: Hunan kexue jishu.

Ma Jixing. 2005. *Chutu wangyi gu yiji yanjiu* 出土亡佚古醫籍研究 [*Study of Excavated Lost Medical Records*]. Beijing: Zhongyi guji.

Mawangdui Han mu boshu zhengli xiaozu 馬王堆漢墓帛書整理小組 [Committee for Organizing the Mawangdui Han Tomb Silk Books], ed. 1985. *Mawangdui Han mu boshu (si)* 馬王堆漢墓帛書(肆) [*Mawangdui Han Tomb Silk Texts*, Vol. 4]. Beijing: Wenwu.

Mcleod, Katrina C. D. & Robin D. S. Yates. 1981. "Forms of Ch'in Law: An Annotated Translation of the *Feng-chen shi*." *Harvard Journal of Asiatic Studies* 41.1: 111–163.

Needham, Joseph. 2000. Nathan Sivin, ed. *Science and Civilisation in China*, Vol. 6. Cambridge: Cambridge University Press.

Perkins, Franklin. 2013. "The Spontaneous Generation of the Human in the 'Heng Xian'." *Dao: A Journal of Comparative Philosophy* 12.2: 225–240.

Raphals, Lisa. 2013. *Divination and Prediction in Early China and Ancient Greece*. Cambridge: Cambridge University Press.

Raphals, Lisa. 2019. "Body and Mind in the Guodian Manuscripts." In Shirley Chan, ed., *Dao Companion to the Excavated Guodian Bamboo Manuscripts*. Dordrecht: Springer, 239–257.

Raphals, Lisa. 2020. "Chinese Philosophy and Chinese Medicine." *The Stanford Encyclopedia of Philosophy* (Winter ed.), ed. Edward N. Zalta. https://plato.stanford.edu/entries/chinese-phil-medicine/ (accessed March 18, 2023).

Raz, Gil. 2014. "Birthing the Self: Metaphor and Transformation in Medieval Daoism." In Jia Jinhua, Kang Xiaofei, & Yao Ping, eds., *Gendering Chinese Religion: Subject, Identity, and Body*. Albany: State University of New York Press, 183–200.

Riegel, Jeffrey. 2012–13. "Curing the Incurable." *Early China* 35–36: 225–246.

Ruan Yuan 阮元, ed. 1987. *Zhouli zhushu* 周禮注疏 [Commentaries on the *Zhouli*]. *Shisan jing zhushu fu jiaokan ji* 十三經注疏附校勘記 [*Collated Notes and Commentaries on the Thirteen Classics*], Vol. 1. Beijing: Zhonghua, 631–939. [First published in 1983.]

Shuihudi Qin mu zhujian zhengli xiaozu 睡虎地秦墓竹簡整理小組 [Committee for Organizing the Shuihudi Qin Tomb Bamboo Slips]. 1990. *Shuihudi Qin mu zhujian* 睡虎地秦墓竹簡 [*Shuihudi Qin Tomb Bamboo Slips*]. Beijing: Wenwu.

Sivin, Nathan. 1993. "*Huang ti nei ching* 黃帝內經." In Michael Loewe, ed. *Early Chinese Texts: A Bibliographical Guide*. Berkeley, CA: Society for the Study of Early China and the Institute of East Asian Studies, 196–215.

Sivin, Nathan. 1995. "State, Cosmos, and Body in the Last Three Centuries B.C." *Harvard Journal of Asiatic Studies* 55.1: 5–37.

Sivin, Nathan. 2017. "Sun Simiao on Medical Ethics: 'The Perfect Integrity of the Great Physician' from Prescriptions worth a Thousand in Gold." In C. Pierce Salguero, ed., *Buddhism and Medicine: An Anthology of Premodern Sources*. New York: Columbia University Press, 538–542.

Smith, Hilary. 2008. "Understanding the *Jiaoqi* Experience: The Medical Approach to Illness in Seventh-Century China." Star Gazing, Firephasing, and Healing in China: Essays in Honor of Nathan Sivin. *Asia Major*, 3rd Series 21.1: 273–292.

Sommer, Deborah. 2008. "Boundaries of the *Ti* Body." *Asia Major*, 3rd Series 21.1: 293–324.

Song, Zhenhao 宋鎮豪. 1995. "Shangdai de wuyi jiaohe hu yiliao suxin" 商代的巫醫校合和醫療俗信 [Shang Magical Medicine and Medical Healing Beliefs]. *Huaxia kaogu* 華夏考古 [*Chinese Archaeology*] 1995.1: 77–13.

Strickmann, Michel. 2002. *Chinese Magical Medicine*. Stanford, CA: Stanford University Press.

Takashima, Ken-ichi. 2010. *Studies of Fascicle Three of Inscriptions from the Yin Ruins*. 2 vols. Institute of History and Philology, Academia Sinica Special Publications No. 107 A, B. Taipei: Academia Sinica.

Tessenow, Hermann & Paul U. Unschuld. 2008. *A Dictionary of the Huang Di nei jing su wen*. Berkeley: University of California Press.

Tian Tian 田天. 2017. "Beida cang Qin jian *Yifang zachao* chushi" 北大藏秦簡《醫方雜抄》初識 [Preliminary Discussion of the Qin Era Bamboo *Yifang zachao* Stored at Beijing University]. *Beijing daxue xuebao* 北京大學學報 [Peking University Academic Journal] 2017.5: 52–57.

Unschuld, Paul U. 1985. *Medicine in China: A History of Ideas*. Berkeley, University of California Press.

Unschuld, Paul U. 2000. *Medicine in China: Historical Artifacts and Images*. Munich: Prestel.

Unschuld, Paul U. 2003. *Huang Di New Jing Su Wen: Nature, Knowledge, Imagery in an Ancient Chinese Medical Text*. Berkeley: University of California Press.

Unschuld, Paul U., trans. 2016a. *Huang Di nei jing ling shu: The Ancient Classic on Needle Therapy*. Berkeley: University of California Press.

Unschuld, Paul U., trans. 2016b. *Nan jing: The Classic of Difficult Issues*. Berkeley: University of California Press.

Unschuld, Paul U. & Hermann Tessenow with Zheng Jinsheng, trans. 2011. *Huang Di nei jing su wen: An Annotated Translation of Huang Di's Inner Classic – Basic Questions*, 2 vols. Berkeley: University of California Press.

Wang Guiyuan 王貴元. 2007. "Zhoujiatai Qin mu jiandu shidu buzheng" 周家台秦墓簡牘釋讀補正 [Added Corrections to the Interpretation of Zhoujiatai Qin Tomb Bamboo and Wooden Slips]. May 8, http://m.bsm.org.cn/?qinjian/4778.html (accessed March 18, 2023).

Wang Qixian 王奇賢 & Zhang Xiancheng 張顯成. 2015. "Chutu san she yi jiandu yanjiuzong" 出土散涉醫簡研究綜 [Summary of Unearthed Scattered Medical Bamboo Slips]. *Guji zhengli yanjiu xuekan* 古籍整理研究學刊 [*Journal for the Study of Ancient Records*] 2015.6: 179–185.

Wang Shuhe 王叔和 (210–285, aka Wang Xi 熙). 2020. *The Pulse Classic. Translation of the* Mai Jing *by Yang Shou-zhong*, 15th ed. Portland, OR: Black Poppy, 2020. [First published in 1997.]

Wang Shumin. 2005. "A General Survey of Medical Works cpmtaomed om the Dunhuang Medical Manuscripts." In Vivienne Lo & Christopher Cullen, eds. *Medieval Chinese Medicine: The Dunhuang Medical Manuscripts*. London: Routledge, 45–58.

Wang Shumin, with Penelope Barrett. 2005. *Abstracts of the Medical Manuscripts from Dunhuang*. London: Curzon. http://idp.bl.uk/database/oo_cat.a4d?shortref=WangShumin_2005&catno=7.2 (accessed March 7, 2021).

Wang Xianshen 王先慎, ed. 1991. *Hanfeizi jijie* 韓非子集解 [Collected Exegeses of *Hanfeizi*]. In *Zhuzi jicheng* 諸子集成 [*Collection of Masters*]. Shanghai: Shanghai shudian, 1986, 1991 rpt. Vol. 5.

Wang Yitong 王一童. 2019. "Laoguanshan Han mu Tianhui yijian *liushi bingfanf he qitangfa* de neiron tedian yu xueshu yuanliu yanjiu" 老官山漢墓天回醫見《六十病方和齊湯法》的內容特點與學術源流研究 [The Contents and Origins of the *Liushi bingfang he Jitang fa* from the Laoguanshan Han Tomb in Tianhui]. Chengdu zhongyiyao daxue 成都中醫藥大學 PhD dissertation, Chengdu University of Chinese Medicine.

Wilms, Sabine. 2005. "'Ten Times More Difficult to Treat': Female Bodies in Medical Texts from Early Imperial China." *Nan nü* 7.2: 74–107.

Wilms, Sabine. 2013. *Venerating the Root, Part 1: Translation of Sun Simiao's Volume on Pediatrics in the Bei Ji Qian Jin Yao Fang*. Corbet, OR: Happy Goat.

Wilms, Sabine. 2015. *Venerating the Root, Part 2: Translation of Sun Simiao's Volume on Pediatrics in the Bei Ji Qian Jin Yao Fang*. Corbet, OR: Happy Goat.

Wuhan jianbo yanjiu zhongxin 武漢簡帛研究中心 & Henansheng wenwu kaogu yanjiusuo 河南省文物考古研究所 [Wuhan Bamboo and Silk Research Center & Henan Provincial Relic and Archaeology Institute], ed. 2013. *Chudi chutu Zhanguo jiance heji (er): Geling Zhanguo zhujian, Changtaiguan Chumu zhujian* 楚地出土戰國簡冊合集(二):葛陵戰國竹簡,長臺關楚墓竹簡 [*Warring States Bamboo Texts Excavated from the Chu Region: Vol. 2: Geling Warring States Bamboo Slips, Changtaiguan Chu Bamboo Slips*]. Beijing: Wenwu.

Xie Minghong 謝明宏. 2018. "Liye Qin jian, "Zhoujiatai Qin jian, Beida cang Qin jian suojian yi jian jishi ji xiangguan wenti yanjiu" 里耶秦簡, 周家台秦簡, 北大藏秦簡所見醫簡集釋及相關問題研究 [Interpretations and Issues with the Qin Era Medical Bamboo Texts from Liye, Zhoujiatai, and Beijing University]. MA thesis, Wuhan University.

Yan Changgui 晏昌貴. 2004. "Tianxingguan 'bushi jidao' jian shiwen jijiao" 天星觀'卜筮祭禱'簡釋文輯校 [Interpretations of the Tianxingguan "Divination and Sacrificial" Bamboo Text]. In Ding Sixin 丁四新, ed. *Chudi jianbo sixiang yanjiu (er)* 楚地簡帛思想研究(二) [*The Thought of Chu Region Bamboo and Silk Texts*, Vol. 2]. Wuhan: Hubei jiaoyu, 265–298.

Yan Yiping 嚴一萍. 1951. *Yin qi zhiyi* 殷契徵醫 [Seeking Medical Help in the Yin Records]. In *Yan Yiping quanji* 嚴一萍全集 [*Collected Writings of Yan Yiping*]. Taibei: Yiwen, 1991.

Yang, Dolly. 2018. "Prescribing 'Guiding and Pulling': The Institutionalization of Therapeutic Exercise in Sui China (581–618 CE)." PhD dissertation, University College London.

Yang Hua 楊華. 2003. "Chutu rishu yu Chu di de jibing zhanbu" 出土日書與楚地的疾病占卜 [Excavated Daybooks and Chu Regional Illness Divination]. *Wuhan daxue xuebao* 武漢大學學報 [Wuhan University Academic Journal] 56.5: 564–570.

Yang, Yong & Miranda Brown. 2017. "The Wuwei Medical Manuscripts: A Brief Introduction and Translation." *Early China* 40: 241–302.

Yu Yue 于越. 2015. "Qin Chu jian bingming yanjiu" 秦楚簡病名研究 [The Names of Ailments in Qin and Chu Bamboo Slips]. 北京中醫藥大學 MA thesis, Beijing University of Chinese Medicine.

Zhang Chaoyang 張朝陽. 2016. "Zhongguo yi faxian zuizao gu yifang: Liye Qin jian zhi yifang jian lüekao" 中國已發現最早醫方: 里耶秦簡之醫方簡略考 [China's Earliest Prescriptions: Liye Qin Bamboo Slip Recipes]. *Tangdu xuekan* 唐都學刊 [*Journal of Tangdu*] 2016.5: 69–74.

Zhang, Hanmo. 2013. "Enchantment, Charming, and the Notion of *Femme Fatale* in Early Chinese Historiography." *Asian Medicine* 8: 249–294.

Zhang Ji (Zhang Zhong-Jing). 2014. *Shang Han Lun (On Cold Damage)*, trans. Craig Mitchell, Feng Ye, & Nigel Wiseman. Taos, NM: Paradigm Publications. [First published in 1997.]

Zhang Ji (Zhang Zhong-Jing). 2013. *Jin Gui Yao Lüe (Essential Prescriptions of the Golden Cabinet)*. Translation by Nigel Wiseman & Sabine Wilms. Taos, NM: Paradigm Publications. [First published in 2000.]

Zhang Shibin & Paul U. Unschuld, eds. 2015. *Dictionary of the Ben Cao Gang Mu, Vol. 1: Chinese Historical Illness Terminology*. Berkeley: University of California Press.

Zhang Wei 張煒. 1998. "Jiaguwen zhong de renti ji shengli renshi" 甲骨文中的人體及生理認識 [Awareness of the Human Body and Physiology in Oracle

Bone Texts]. *Zhongyi wenxian zazhi* 中醫文獻雜誌 [Magazine of Chinese Medical Texts] 1998.1: 12–13.

Zheng Jinsheng, Nalini Kirk, Paul D. Buell, & Paul U. Unschuld, eds. 2018. *Dictionary of the Ben Cao Gang Mu, Vol. 3: Persons and Literary Sources.* Berkeley: University of California Press.

Zhongguo shehui kexueyuan kaogu yanjiusuo Hebeisheng wenwu guanlichu 中國社會科學院考古研究所河北省文物管理處 [Hebei Provincial Relics Administration of the Chinese Academy of Social Science Archaeological Research Institute], ed. 1980. *Mancheng Han mu fajue baogao* 滿城漢墓發掘報告 [*Excavation Report on the Han Tombs at Mancheng*]. 2 vols. Beijing: Wenwu.

Cambridge Elements ≡

Ancient East Asia

Erica Fox Brindley

Pennsylvania State University

Erica Fox Brindley is Professor and Head in the Department of Asian Studies at Pennsylvania State University. She is the author of three books, co-editor of several volumes, and the recipient of the ACLS Ryskamp Fellowship and Humboldt Fellowship. Her research focuses on the history of the self, knowledge, music, and identity in ancient China, as well as on the history of the Yue/Viet cultures from southern China and Vietnam.

Rowan Kimon Flad

Harvard University

Rowan Kimon Flad is the John E. Hudson Professor of Archaeology in the Department of Anthropology at Harvard University. He has authored two books and over 50 articles, edited several volumes, and served as editor of Asian Perspectives. His archaeological research focuses on economic and ritual activity, interregional interaction, and technological and environmental change, in the late Neolithic and early Bronze Ages of the Sichuan Basin and the Upper Yellow River valley regions of China.

About the Series

Elements in Ancient East Asia contains multi-disciplinary contributions focusing on the history and culture of East Asia in ancient times. Its framework extends beyond anachronistic, nation-based conceptions of the past, following instead the contours of Asian sub-regions and their interconnections with each other. Within the series there are five thematic groups: 'Sources', which includes excavated texts and other new sources of data; 'Environments', exploring interaction zones of ancient East Asia and long-distance connections; 'Institutions', including the state and its military; 'People', including family, gender, class, and the individual and 'Ideas', concerning religion and philosophy, as well as the arts and sciences. The series presents the latest findings and strikingly new perspectives on the ancient world in East Asia.

Cambridge Elements ⹀

Ancient East Asia

Elements in the Series